D1536457

"Alternately enlightening and enraging, *Bent out of Shape* made me look at the world of work in a whole new way. Messing deftly illustrates how gender differences rooted in both biology and social roles have been treated with a toxic mixture of sexism, shame, and secrecy by businesses, governments, and unions, resulting in untold costs in illness, injury, and misery. *Bent out of Shape* shows us that efforts to enforce workplace equality by ignoring gender differences have not resulted in true workplace equity. Advocating for better data, design, and policy, Messing draws on her decades of experience grappling with workplace inequality to propose solutions that would lead to healthier, safer, and more respectful workplaces for everyone."

LESLIE KERN, author of *Feminist City: A Field Guide*

"A compelling and important book about the health of women in the workplace. I have followed Karen Messing's work for years, and hers is a unique voice, focused on working women, using feminist research tools and theories, but striving always to understand how the social and the biological are interlaced. Want to improve working conditions and on-the-job health for women? Read this book!"

ANNE FAUSTO-STERLING, professor emerita of biology and gender studies, Brown University

"Once more, Dr. Karen Messing succeeds at captivating us with her beautiful writing; her well-crafted, thought-provoking anecdotes taken from her firsthand experience as an advocate for women's rights; and her accessible use of the latest science on sex and gender issues in occupational health. Messing's books are essential in bridging the gaps between generations of researchers and advocates for women's health. I will be sure to add this to the list of recommended readings for my class and for my non-academic friends as well."

> JULIE CÔTÉ, professor and department chair, Department of Kinesiology and Physical Education, McGill University

"It may seem somehow wrong to say that a book called *Bent out of Shape* is a pleasure to read. However, I did find it a pleasure to read this provocative, complex, self-reflective, and witty analysis of the need to overcome the shame related to women's bodies at work, as well as the importance of solidarity in addressing the contradictory pressures to recognize the specificity and diversity of bodies while working for equity. Informed by scientific evidence at the same time as it critiques the lack of evidence and makes it all accessible to the broadest audience, the book clearly establishes the need to take bodies into account in all labour processes. It should be compulsory reading for everyone, manager and worker alike."

> PAT ARMSTRONG, distinguished research professor of sociology, York University

"A crucially important book for the growing field of sex and gender science. It describes the science of the female body as it meets the world of work and documents the many clashes of sex and gender that result in women's occupational injury. In asking a range of important questions about how to fix sexist and damaging occupational practices and policies, Messing challenges all of us: unions, management, consumers, policy makers, women, and men to speak up and lose our reticence, whether it be based on shame or desperation, ignorance or oppression. An important read."

> LORRAINE GREAVES, senior investigator, Centre of
> Excellence for Women's Health

"Messing's exploration into the gendered impact of work is illuminating. From rates of workplace injury to spaces designed explicitly for men, she offers an important critique of how the physical plays an important role in maintaining the patriarchy."

> NORA LORETO, author of *Take Back the Fight: Organizing Feminism for the Digital Age*

BENT OUT OF SHAPE

SHAME, SOLIDARITY, AND WOMEN'S BODIES AT WORK

KAREN MESSING

BETWEEN THE LINES
TORONTO

Bent out of Shape
© 2021 Karen Messing

First published in 2021 by
Between the Lines
401 Richmond Street West, Studio 281
Toronto, Ontario · M5V 3A8 · Canada
1-800-718-7201 · www.btlbooks.com

Cataloguing in Publication information available from
Library and Archives Canada · ISBN 9781771135412

Cover design by Michael DeForge
Text design by DEEVE

Printed in Canada

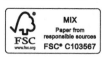

We acknowledge for their financial support of our publishing activities: the
Government of Canada; the Canada Council for the Arts; and the Government
of Ontario through the Ontario Arts Council, the Ontario Book Publishers Tax
Credit program, and Ontario Creates.

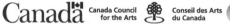 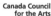 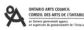

CONTENTS

PREFACE

I have always been active, but never a real athlete. In grade six, I was happy to be the third-fastest girl runner in my class, mostly because my growth spurt came early so I was the tallest. I did my best for our relay team at the city-wide finals, but we came in last. So I was delighted when I realized that I was pretty good at the standing broad jump. On a good day, I could jump 71 inches (1.8 metres), better than everyone in my grade, girls and boys. I practised jumping all the time and dreamed of winning at the next city competition.

My dream dissolved when my mother spoke to me, clearly an emissary from on high. "Your father is worried about you. He is afraid that all that jumping is bad for your female organs." At eleven, I hadn't thought a lot about my female organs; in fact I wasn't too sure what they were talking about. And, in 1954, I wasn't about to ask them. But my mother's remark was enough to get me imagining all these insides that looked like chicken livers and gizzards, hanging somewhere in my body from long strings, bouncing around and bumping into each other. I began to think of my body as less fit. My enthusiasm for jumping waned and I didn't win the competition. For the next few years, I carried with me the image of the livers on strings, and didn't jump around much. (You will notice that I went through all this alone, never discussed my insides with my girlfriends, never shared my concerns with my gym teachers—more about this shame later.)

Nine years later, during my first pregnancy, I was again faced with a lot of outside opinions on my body. My tummy seemed to encourage passersby to be generous with their criticism. The new lot of commentators were worried because I continued to bicycle to work. I was going to fall and have a miscarriage, I was going to hurt my baby, I was going to bring on a premature delivery. This time I went and got professional advice. My obstetrician said not to worry; one of his patients had fallen out of a second-storey window during her fifth month, with no consequences to the fetus. I stayed on my bike, kept away from open windows, and stopped worrying about my female organs for a while. But I had become irretrievably aware that my body was flawed and subject to criticism from anyone passing by.

Studying women's biology

I entered graduate school in biology in 1968 when my sons were five and two, over the objections of professors who felt being a mother in itself disqualified me from doing a doctorate. My (male) supervisors fought to get me in, and I was content to be there. I could do interesting experiments and read articles on cells and DNA at the medical school library. Once in a while I strayed onto the physiology shelves, and there I stumbled across a book with the Olympic records for running and jumping. I was happy to learn that many pregnant women had competed in the Olympics, with no consequences to the fetus or, as far as I could tell, to their female organs.[1] I became curious about women's biology, although it was far from my master's thesis on fruit fly heredity. Occasionally an article on human sex chromosomes slid itself into the pile of articles about flies.

Still a student in 1972, I got a call from a group of professors at the Université du Québec à Montréal (UQAM) who wanted to establish courses in women's studies. They had been able to negotiate one course, to be taught in the history department. But they were ambitious: they wanted to have several different versions of the course, one on women and economics, another on women and politics, and so on. With the help of Professor Donna Mergler, I took on the women and biology course. This was my first teaching job, rather far removed from my laboratory studies, and challenging, since I had a lot to learn about women's biology and the students kept asking me hard questions. I looked for answers at the library, as graduate students did, but I was dismayed to find that there was little in the scientific literature that would answer the students' questions about menopause, menstrual cramps, body shape, or environmental effects on pregnancy. I muddled along as best I could while continuing the laboratory research that would eventually get me my PhD in genetics.

When I became Dr. Messing, UQAM hired me as a professor. But, as I have described elsewhere,[2] I was enticed out of my laboratory by an agreement between UQAM and three Quebec trade unions that provided resources for research and teaching in occupational health (and other fields). I started to spend a lot of time with low-paid, low-prestige workers, most of them women, who struggled to get me to understand what their work involved. At the same time, one of my colleagues inveigled me onto the professors' union executive by lying about the amount of time involved. I ended up being sent to serve on the women's committee of my union confederation, which, in the late 1970s, was grappling with issues around equality and health protection. What was equal work? Why was women's pay lower than men's? Was it because of physical exertion? Then why would physicians be paid more than cleaners? Should women have to lift as much weight as men to receive equal pay? What if the weights are people who squirm and resist in daycare centres and seniors' residences, should that count extra? Do women and men run an equal risk of health damage from any chemicals? all chemicals? Does pregnancy render women unable to work? at all jobs? Should women be working nights in factories? If not, why do they work nights in hospitals?

I started to think about how workplaces treat biological differences between women and men. Should our dreams really be limited by our bodies? Do we have to be the same as men to be equal?

People thought I should have answers to some of these questions because I understood how genes and chromosomes worked. I did know that people usually have forty-six chromosomes but that biological women and men almost always differ by a single chromosome. Women and men have twenty-two pairs of chromosomes that are grossly the same, but the twenty-third pair is different: 99 percent of people designated as women have two big X chromosomes, while 99 percent of men have one big X and one tiny Y. Knowing that didn't help me much, though—I couldn't find anything in the genetics literature to explain the links between having an X or Y chromosome and job segregation by sex. No one had unearthed a gene for any trait qualifying people for truck driving (most common men's job) or being an office worker or teacher (most common women's jobs). They still haven't.

Some penetrating questions from hospital cleaners led me to seek training in ergonomics, a science that seeks to understand work and make it healthier. I then spent years working in partnership with union women's committees and occupational health committees to study the work of bank tellers, primary school teachers, cleaners, and many other women.

From shame to solidarity

For a few years, my department grumpily allowed me to continue teaching my biology and women course in addition to what they called my "disciplinary" courses in genetics. As if women's biology wasn't *real* biology.

One year I showed the 1977 film *À notre santé* (To Our Health), about the women's self-help movement, produced by health activists in Quebec and Italy.[3] I had meant to use it to discuss that movement's view of women's biology, since their bible, *Our Bodies, Ourselves,* had just come out in French as *Notre corps, nous-mêmes.* But the discussion got derailed. After the film, the all-female class was silent for a while, and then a tall, young woman said the film was ugly. It turned out she was referring to a couple of shots of women's external genitals. The students spent the whole rest of the class sharing how much they hated their bodies. Everyone, all these beautiful young women, felt ugly everywhere. My reaction? It was hard for me to guide the conversation because I felt the same, except that in my eyes they were all beautiful and I was the only ugly one. Not to mention my unthinkable genitals. It was a revelation to all of us, I think, to realize that we were all ashamed, very deeply ashamed, of our bodies. And ourselves.

I think some of this shame came from a double bind about sexual aggression. There is no right way to be a young woman. As the #MeToo movement has pointed out, if we don't smile at everyone no matter what, we are bitches, but if we do, we are sluts. I was ashamed about the boys who lied about me being "easy" when I was fourteen, too humiliated to explain myself to the adults who believed them. Ashamed when a camp director attacked me while walking in the woods when I was fifteen. When a clever law student tricked, argued, and pressured me into performing sexual services when I was sixteen, changing forever the way I felt about men's bodies. When a Harvard lecturer responded to my question about economic theory with a farfetched analogy about my "reproductive capacity," making the other students laugh and shutting me up in class for the next two years. Shame about the exhibitionists, the guys who grabbed at my body parts in Paris and Montreal, the young kid in Athens who took advantage of my carrying a huge, heavy box to feel my breasts. Facing the unrelenting pressure to do this, that, and the other thing. With a smile.

The shame at giving in, and at smiling, was silent. Just as I had kept quiet about the livers and gizzards, I never told anyone at all about the sexual attacks for a good fifty years, because I was sure I would be blamed. As I often blamed other women.

Research on women's jobs

It took a while for me to see the connections between the shame in my biology class and what I was hearing, and not hearing, from the working women: the long silences when I asked whether the women were at ease in their previously all-male ghettos, nervous denial if I asked whether they were bothered by sexist jokes, reluctant admission that they found it hard to keep lifting patients, downplayed desperation about getting to work on time after a baby joined the family. As often as not, it was their male colleagues who were able to tell me about some of the injustices—about a bank manager who let male clerks, but not women, work with their backs to the public, about sexual harassment of women cleaners. An immigrant man in a clothing factory said it best:

> Sometimes they have some problems with the machine
> or the production line, you know, how to manage, or they
> have some problems with co-workers, they compete, and

some bullies. They cannot say. . . . I know some Chinese persons, some ladies feel hurt in their heart, they cannot say. They just keep silent because they cannot say.[4]

I don't think the man was referring only to the women's limited command of English and French.

From 1993 to 2012, our joint research effort with women's committees in three union confederations tried to make the "hurt in their heart" visible. In fact, that is the name we gave our program: *l'Invisible qui fait mal*, or The Invisible That Hurts. Through our research, I have come to think that women workers need to combat our shame about our "different" bodies head-on. We need to dare to direct attention to the risks in our work, combatting all attempts to blame us for getting injured. And, above all, we need to develop ways to protect each other while we struggle together to adapt the workplace to our bodies and our lives.

I have come to believe that some of our failures to attain equality and health at work come from obstacles we haven't been facing and don't like to talk about—such as biological and social differences between women and men. I have seen (and been among) working women choked to silence by shame about being physically weaker, about menstruating, about needing to get to the daycare centre on time, about hot flashes, and I've realized that we need to think hard about the costs of our silence and talk with each other about solutions.

I have been forced to re-examine not only my personal, private experiences with aggression and shaming, but also our professional successes and failures. How does solidarity relate to ergonomic interventions in the workplace? Can it help us to improve women's health and safety at work? Is it ridiculous to try to apply solidarity to ergonomic interventions to improve women's work, and even to the science behind our interventions?

In the workplace, women have to deal with our bodies being considered "second bodies"—different, abnormal, inferior in size and strength. When we enter the job market, our jobs are often "second jobs"—supposedly easier, requiring fewer abilities, and worth less pay. Employers tell us that any mom who is well organized and insists on working for pay should be able to make it in to work on time every single day while keeping her "second" family role invisible. No mom could possibly believe that, but, like the immigrant workers, we "cannot say." And our work-related health problems are accorded little importance, since they are considered imaginary (depression, anxiety), resulting from weakness (musculoskeletal disorders), weird (associated with pregnancy or menopause), or yucky (menstrual disorders). This lack of respect for women's specific needs ends up making it nearly impossible for us to demand equality and health protection at the same time.

How to change this? Women need to name the aggression we face and hold responsible those who attack us. We need to name and combat the shame we feel when we are attacked for being women. We need to stand together to make real changes in the systems that support our attackers. Our network of powerful, beautiful feminist ergonomists is struggling to combat shame with solidarity, and I will describe our struggles and what we have learned.

Important stuff I won't be talking about very much

I am only going to say this once, but it's important. Men are also oppressed at work, have unrecognized work accidents and illnesses, and have to battle with unsympathetic employers and government agencies. Many (most?) men do not conform fully with gender and sex stereotypes and suffer from ill-adapted work sites. This book is about women at work because I have mainly done research on women's jobs and because it is more often women (and gender non-conforming men) who experience a forced choice between gender equality and their health.

A friend of mine warned me early on that my book shouldn't only talk about cis women. But I have to say that, in the unionized, low-paid workplaces where we have done our observations, trans and non-binary women have not been visible, just as gender non-conforming men have not been visible. I'm not saying there weren't any, just that they were not visible. And my major message in the book can only be based on what I have seen and heard in the workplace. Yes, most physical, social, and psychological characteristics of women and men overlap; yes, women and men and everyone else should be able to access all jobs. But—there are areas where there is little or no overlap in physical characteristics, where many women (and a few others) are disproportionately affected by the fact that workplaces were designed for the average XY body. Not only spaces but also tools, schedules, and work teams were designed in a binary world where European, upper-class, cis men dominate. So the physical reality of most women (body shape, strengths and weaknesses, menstruation, pregnancy, menopause, double workday, likelihood of sexual assault) has been excluded. And (cis and other) women find it hard to fight for workplace adaptation, not only because of power imbalance, lack of a voice, ignorance, and sexism, but also because any request for change is seen as disqualification for the job.

As far as gender (social roles) as opposed to sex (biological differences) is concerned, my message has to do with the sexism experienced by all who identify / are identified by others as women. Women in the workplace are confined to certain jobs, tasks, movements, and behaviours and suffer the consequences.

My apologies also go to racialized and immigrant workers, because I haven't had much opportunity to observe their work, either. Professor Stephanie Premji did her PhD work with us at the request of a union with many immigrant workers, and she has gone on to learn a lot about immigrant workers' occupational health. I recommend her books and articles.[5]

PART I.
SHAME AND THE
WORKPLACE

1.
THE THIRD HOUR

My research collaborators and I were in a small room without
windows, and it was seven in the evening. The other five
women in the room had worked all that day as communications technicians, responsible for repairing or installing material in
homes, businesses, and construction sites. They set up phone lines
and solved problems with static and internet connections. We had
invited them because the union women's service wanted to know
how to keep women from leaving this job, where they were a small
and diminishing minority (30 out of 1,273 workers in the company
in Quebec). And the women's service wanted to know how to help
women stay in non-traditional jobs, because the problem of attri-
tion was general.[1]

Five of the ten women based in Montreal came to the meeting,
after their workday had finished. Although they had seen each other
around, the women had never been together as a group. We asked
them what they did at work, whether it affected their health, and
whether they wanted to bring up any issues about being women at
this job. At first, no one had much to say. They didn't see why they
were meeting with us—what was the point? They had no particular

problems to tell us about, nor were they treated any differently from their male colleagues. Occasionally, customers would refuse to let them enter their house or insult them because they were women. They had been trying to deal with these problems on their own. Chantal[2] was the most vocal, but she said she had no complaints. Her co-workers were fine, her foreman treated her well, she liked her job. Sophie mentioned that she didn't like all the sexist jokes, so she objected to them. We asked questions from our list, but Josée, Barbara, and Johanne had nothing in particular they wanted to share.

During the second hour, the room started to feel smaller and a little more unsettled. Chantal told us she had asked her foreman in confidence to send another technician to service a customer who had put the moves on her, but the foreman lost no time before telling everyone about her problem, which then became a source of general amusement. Why then had the same foreman been so careful to keep it quiet when her colleague Patrick had been cruised by a male customer? But, she said, it didn't really *bother* her, she just kept on doing her job. Several of the women had trouble with tools and wondered why smaller sizes weren't available, but, they said, it wasn't a *serious* problem. Johanne had asked several times for a smaller tool belt but it never arrived. She said she could do the job with the big belt, but it weighed over three kilograms and hurt her hips. We asked whether adding a cross-chest harness would make it easier to carry the tools, since the weight would be shared between shoulders and hips.

Everyone laughed. "Yeah sure, we're going to have a strap coming across our front pushing our breasts out—we spend our whole day trying to make them forget we're women." The room took a deep breath.

And then, during the third hour, we heard what the job was really like. All the women (except for Johanne, whose husband worked with her so she was usually spared) had developed different strategies to deal with the sexist jokes and insulting remarks. One "built a wall," never engaging in social contacts. Several had learned to laugh or even engage in repartee, but they found it tiring. Sophie, the feminist, was so weary from the constant battles for respect that she was thinking of leaving (she did leave the company two years later).

They told us about their battles with the ladders, which each had waged alone. The company had ladders in three sizes: 24, 26, and 28 feet long. The ladders were heavy and awkward to carry, quite hard to install on top of the trucks, especially for smaller people. In the Montreal area, only 24-foot ladders were thought to be necessary, so in theory all trucks were equipped with the smaller ladders that were somewhat easier to handle. But in fact, often only 26- or 28-foot ladders were available. Each of the women had tried to get her foreman to order more of the smaller ladders or at least to reserve the smaller ones for them, but this hadn't worked.

As we got further into the third hour, we heard more stories: other wrong-sized tools, verbal attacks, colleagues who wouldn't stop harassing, colleagues who refused to work with them and actively tried to get them fired. It was as if the women felt they should take these problems in their stride, as if the problems were the price of "invading" male territory. But by this time, the women in the room had realized that they all faced the same obstacles and they became able, even eager, to share their challenges and think about solutions. A real solidarity moment for all of us.

We got the employer to allow us to observe the technicians' work. With a student, Marie-Christine Thibault, my colleague Céline Chatigny and I observed the work of three female and four male communications technicians for a total of 123 hours.[3] We observed women and men wiring panels in all sorts of conditions: outside, inside, in pleasant and horrible weather. They spent a lot of

5

time alone driving vans from one work site to another. The women sometimes had to negotiate entry into private homes, despite the residents' insistence that they wanted a "qualified" (that is, male) technician. They installed new wiring and fixed old installations. Technicians discussed and solved problems in informal groups, during breaks or mealtimes. They had to slither into tiny spaces (small women had an advantage) and stretch out to reach high on walls (an advantage for the taller men).

There should have been another woman in our original meeting, but Valérie was home on sick leave. Months later, we learned that she had been raped on the job by another worker, but no one had told us about it, even during the third hour. Our union contacts hadn't told us about Valérie either, even though the rape was probably why we had been asked to do the study. Céline heard from colleagues about Valérie's terrifying experience, and about how unsupportive, even hostile, her foreman, colleagues, and union had been. Although Valerie had immediately called police, no one was "able" to identify the culprit, who had left the scene. This anonymity seemed unlikely, since the man was presumably on someone's payroll, so Valérie suspected male complicity. She went home, suffering from post-traumatic stress disorder. She tried to return to work two days later, but she became afraid of a co-worker assigned to her because his mannerisms reminded her of the aggressor. She asked for a change of assignment, but her foreman just told her to get over it. She was eventually let go after two years at the company, and told us she thought it was because her co-worker didn't want to work with a woman. But, when Céline asked Valérie our standard question about differences in how women and men were treated at work, she was amazed at the response: "There's no problem, no difference, men and women are the same." We could only think that Valérie had diagnosed her rape as a personal, individual problem, possibly due to some weakness or mistake of her own.

When Céline interviewed Sophie, she heard more about the possibility that women and men might not be treated the same. Sophie, the only worker who openly identified as a feminist, had tried hard to keep the men from making sexist jokes. She told us, sadly, that she had felt she'd made progress and was even accepted as "one of the guys," until one morning in the restaurant where the technicians gathered to plan their work, share problems, and enjoy each other's company:

I don't know what started it. The technician opposite me, talking to the waitress: "Damn bitch!" and stuff like that. I reacted "Pardon me!" . . . I looked at the waitress and I said, "Excuse me, but I wouldn't wait on people who talk to me like that." [The male technician answered,] "Ah! It's a joke! You should stick with us guys!" I said, "Sorry, but that's just [not] good manners, talking to someone like that, I totally don't find that funny, not at all." The guys all stood up at once. I swear, there were ten of them at the table. [He said,] "Yes, okay, it's fine. I think we'll all go now." They all left [to sit at another table]; I finished my toast all by myself.[4]

After that, Sophie always ate breakfast alone, deprived not only of companionship but of an important source of technical know-how and help in solving problems. In fact, we noted that all the women were eating alone, set apart from their male colleagues.

This sad story, and others the technicians told us, left us feeling ashamed of our own inability to help. The local union seemed to be uninterested in the women's problems, and the women's service of the union confederation didn't seem to have any influence on them. After our initial meeting with the women technicians, there was no local follow-up and none of the technicians wanted to form a women's committee, possibly because they didn't want to make themselves any more visible as women.

Discrimination and health

We were interested in health effects of the technicians' work, so we examined their registry of work accidents. We found that women had many more work accidents than men: about three times as many accidents as men on a per employee basis, over a four-year period (Figure 1.1).

This is not unusual. We later found similar results in landscaping, another non-traditional workplace.[5] The US Army has found a

Figure 1.1 Accidents per employee in telecommunications

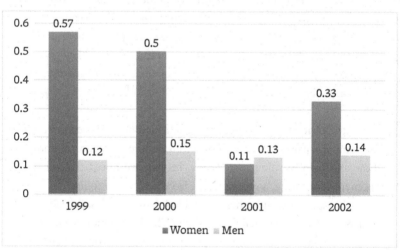

Source: Karen Messing, Ana Maria Seifert, and Vanessa Couture, "Les femmes dans les métiers non-traditionnels : Le général, le particulier et l'ergonomie," *Travailler* 15 (2006), 131–48.

significantly higher rate of injury among female soldiers,[6] and health and safety authorities in Quebec report that, when women are in the same industries as men, women generally have a higher rate of accidents and injuries.[7] In heavy manufacturing, women have 36 percent more injuries than men.[8] Among the potential explanations: the women could be more likely to report accidents; the equipment and training could be ill adapted; the women could be less experienced; the women could be physically less able to do the job without injury. In the case of our research with the communications technicians, there were not enough women to allow us to distinguish statistically among these possibilities, but we did look into the equipment. Because the women had brought up ladders during our initial meeting, we focused on accidents with ladders.

Work on ladders was the single largest cause of accidents in the registry. For both women and men, 31 percent of accidents involved ladders: climbing them and carrying them. Given that women had proportionately more accidents, this rate of 31 percent meant that women were having a lot of accidents with ladders. Céline and Marie-Christine found a number of problems while observing how the ladders were used. They weighed about 50 kilograms (the weight of a small woman) and had to be carried around on all sorts of surfaces. In the winter, technicians had to carry them through icy alleys, and in spring, through mud. Technicians leaned the ladders against slippery poles and rested them on slick surfaces. While the technicians were climbing the ladders, they were also wearing their heavy tool belts. Céline found that, in general, the size of all this equipment was too big and/or badly proportioned for many women: the ladders were unnecessarily long even when collapsed, the harnesses were too big, the belts were too wide and too heavy. The task of carrying a ladder was harder for all the women.

And training had not been adapted. Women were told to use techniques that just didn't work for shorter, less powerful people with a lower centre of gravity. Carrying the ladders in the recommended position over the shoulder while gripping two rungs a metre apart, close to one end, was impossible for many of the women, the shortest of whom was 1.54 metres (5 feet) tall. The trainers had never been asked to think about how women should carry ladders.

So women were less able to do this job without injury, because no one had thought about how to adapt the job for a wider variety of physical bodies.

Women technicians leave the scene

Three years after we began the study, only two of the original ten women in Montreal were still on the job and they had both had work accidents; two were on sick leave and six were gone. At the provincial level, women had been 16 of the 1,257 technicians; only the two in Montreal were left. When we talked to the union people, this preferential loss of women workers from a non-traditional job turned out to be relatively common. As feminists, we felt sorry that all these women were made to feel like failures when they had tried so hard to do these jobs "just like a man."

We submitted our report to the union confederation. We described the problems and suggested the unions negotiate more appropriate ways to integrate women entering non-traditional jobs, from apprenticeships to supervisor training to changes in tools, equipment, and work methods. The report was returned to us several times in the hope that we would soften it; those at the top of the union hierarchy appeared afraid that the men, a majority at the confederation, would be insulted and angry. Finally, we were invited to present the report to about a hundred union women from various non-traditional workplaces. After Céline presented our results, there was silence. Then, one woman said a few words about her painful experience in a male-dominated workplace, then another woman, then another, as more and more women lined up at the microphone. They told of physical problems with equipment, training issues, and social obstacles to their integration and retention in these jobs. Céline and I felt like crying. Another solidarity moment.

We were touched by the strength, courage, and frankness of the women. Until a very high ranking male member of the union confederation seized the mic. He denounced the "negative atmosphere" and asked for more "positive" contributions. The large room went quiet. The women shut up completely, including those from the women's committee. We ourselves were silent, not wanting to make trouble for the women who had invited us and feeling that it was up to the union members to decide how to treat their elected officials. But I have often wondered whether I should have been more vocal. Céline says she still shivers thinking about the episode.

What should we have done, faced with the women's reluctance to confront the powerful men? Should we be ashamed of our hesitation to defend them? Was a whole roomful of women suffering from shame? From a lack of solidarity? Or just from fear?

Why doesn't the employer respond?

Even if the women's union was slow to defend them, one would think that it would be in the employer's interest to help women be more productive. But company management does not appear to be judged by its ability to manage change for women. In the early 2000s, I was an expert witness in a human rights case brought by a women's advocacy group, Action travail des femmes, against the local gas company. Seven plaintiffs had been refused employment in pipe maintenance. They charged that the pre-employment test and screening process discriminated against women, because the human resources personnel appeared hostile and the tests were not related to the actual requirements of the job. Some of the tests targeted abilities and experience not related to the job but more familiar to men, such as car repair, and women did relatively badly. In 2007, Sophie Brochu became president of the gas company, to much fanfare because she was the first woman and, according to the company, a progressive thinker. Quebeckers often hear her commenting on the social responsibility of companies and on environmental efforts. She likes to mention her activities in support of the advancement of women and improving education in poor communities.[9] So we thought she might weigh in on the side of the women.

But when the human rights tribunal found for the plaintiffs in 2008, the very next year, her gas company appealed, stalling application of the decision for the following three years, when the appeal was definitively rejected.[10]

The gas company was fined and told it had to introduce an affirmative action plan. I don't know whether Brochu had tried to prevent her company from appealing the human rights decision or from pursuing their case against the women. I have not seen any public reaction to the decision from Brochu, and the women's advocacy group never heard from her. In 2017, Brochu accepted the position of spokeswoman on pay equity for the provincial authority on labour standards. In 2020, the Quebec government hired her to head Hydro-Québec, our electricity supplier. It doesn't seem like you have to defend working women if you want to play an important role managing public employees.

Landscaping: a similar experience

As part of the same research program and at the request of a union women's committee, we also examined the work of women in landscaping, members of a different union who were working on private property. This work was physically harder than that of the technicians, and male-female biological differences became even more visible. Women had trouble driving the litter-cleaning machine because the seat was too far from the pedals and the pedals needed to be pushed hard to make them work. Working the levers of the backhoe excavator required a lot of arm strength, and digging holes was hard on the women's backs. Women reported much more chronic pain than men, and as in the previous study, the women had two to three times as many work accidents.

Again, the local union was less than helpful, and again, the employer, headed by a woman, showed no interest in our report. The women working in landscaping were even more distant from one another than in the communications company. Although they saw each other every day, they spoke rarely, and any lesbians who had come out were particularly isolated and subject to homophobic remarks. Isolation was a particular danger at this job because a work accident could happen far from the company headquarters. We observed a worker attacked and stung by bees, quickly succoured by a colleague who applied first aid. We heard about workers falling into deep holes and being quickly covered and suffocated by falling dirt; only an alert colleague could rescue them. Workers needed to be able to count on their colleagues for immediate help, so the isolated women were less protected.

More aggression and denial, by government feminists

While I was doing these studies, a young journalist contacted me because he had a contract with the Quebec ministry responsible for women's affairs. He was to write a brochure on women entering non-traditional jobs. I was happy to collaborate because I had come to hate the cheery government advertisements that encouraged women to "do anything you want" without mentioning the obstacles. Competitions like Chapeau, les filles! (Hats off to girls)[11] inviting young women to enter the trades seemed to me like wolves encouraging Little Red Riding Hood to enter their lair. I wanted to warn the women and see whether the government could develop programs to help them avoid getting eaten.

After I described the biological differences and similarities between women and men, the journalist and I had a long chat about the obstacles our research group had found in our studies and our suggestions for adapting tools and training. I told him about our recommended approaches to male-female relations at work. I wanted to figure out some government policy solutions for the refusal to adapt ladders and tool belts, the mistreatment of Valérie's rape, Sophie's experience in the restaurant, and ours in the union meeting. I thought the alpha males who led the attacks might be hard to re-educate, but I wondered whether the other men couldn't have been encouraged not to follow their example.

The journalist took lots of notes, wrote them up and sent me a draft of his brochure for validation. Lo and behold, I was quoted as a biology expert, saying only that women could do anything men could do. All my analyses and recommendations for change and support for the women were gone. I carefully corrected his text and sent it back, but the ministry published his original version of our interview.

What a disappointment! Actions conceived by women in order to help advance women workers in non-traditional workplaces ended up ineffectual, and the union hierarchy and the government feminists responsible for improving things closed their eyes and plugged their ears.

What aggressions do we need to name?
What shame do we need to combat?

We saw that (1) women were being introduced into jobs where they were a tiny minority without any open consideration of potential social problems or adjustment of training, equipment, or tools; (2) these women faced open hostility as well as thinly veiled efforts at exclusion through sexist jokes and demeaning remarks; (3) the women were in danger of sexual aggression; (4) a union, normally highly involved in defending workers' rights, did not unequivocally support its own women's service in defending these women; and (5) the women did not say openly that they were endangered and actively denied that they suffered discrimination.

This last point is crucial. Why were the women so reluctant to name or even acknowledge the social and physical problems? When we were talking with the communications technicians, women only started to share their experiences during the third hour of our meeting, and even then, they tended to minimize the threats they faced. We have observed this phenomenon of the "third hour" several times since. I came to see an analogy with rape victims, who can take years to acknowledge the damage they have suffered because they are ashamed of what was done to them. The workers can feel that if they were stronger, smarter, nicer, or not too nice, somehow the aggressions wouldn't happen. They try harder and harder until they give up and leave.

The union women's committee involved in the communications study set up an interview with eight women from other local unions, in jobs like truck driver, gardener, mechanic, and welder. Again, it took the women over two hours to be able to start to talk about the problems they experienced. All denied at first that they had any physical or social problems at their jobs. It was only when they started to feel safe that they shared their feelings of defeat and physical and psychological exhaustion. And we found the same story in a different majority-female union confederation. When Jessica Riel was finishing her PhD research with women responsible for secondary-level vocational training in traditionally male jobs, she set up a collective telephone interview to get feedback on her results. She let me listen in: two hours of denial that there were any problems, of insistence that the women were treated as equals by the other teachers. Then, bit by bit, first confiding and then bonding about physical and social problems. It was as if the women needed to hear that they hadn't caused their own misery by making terrible, unforgivably incompetent, individual mistakes, before they could open up. Talking about their experiences for two hours, with our encouragement, helped them let go of their shame and start to support each other. But we had to worry about what would happen next. What would happen to the teachers when each was left alone in her own school, strung out in different towns across the province? Would their union follow through and support them?

Going it alone doesn't work

Some years ago, I was the union representative for the science faculty at UQAM. That meant people came to me with problems. One new professor came to me because she was being sexually harassed and generally mistreated. She had been hired because her previously all-male department had no choice: her research record was outstanding and our women's committee and the women's studies group were scrutinizing all hiring. But the department hated her— she was blocked when she tried to do anything at all, from getting her lab equipped to teaching the courses she had been hired for. And her department chair, a married man, had to be turned away when he showed up at her apartment several times, late at night, "to talk."

Despite all this, she insisted that her being a woman was irrelevant to her problems. She thought the men were mean, not sexist or predatory. She didn't want the women's committee to get involved; it would only make things worse. She wanted me to suggest some other way to solve her problems, although clearly, it was not accidental that she had come to me, a known feminist. But she didn't want any official union involvement, either. I had no advice that she felt able to take, and she eventually went on stress leave. While she was away, her department was dissolved for general incompetence, and she never came back.

This episode taught me something. Most of us are extremely scared of naming gender discrimination. The professor, like the communications technicians, didn't want to admit that she faced discrimination at work because the problem would then become public and "political" and thus too big to handle by her usual technique of quietly proving her competence. To gain access to non-traditional jobs, all these women had overcome many obstacles, one by one, and their patience and persistence had worked for them. They had encountered insults and opposition before, and they had just gritted their teeth and stuck it out. The communications technicians had gotten good, well-paying jobs, and the scientist had gotten research grants and an enviable university position. Why not just carry on?

But unfortunately, single combat only got them so far, as we can see from the large number of women who got sick and/or left their jobs. Fundamental change had to come if they were to stay on. Change not only in the social relations at work, but in workplace training, tools, and equipment, in record keeping, in accident prevention, and in union action. But for this to happen, the groundbreaking women would have to admit that their situation was not exactly the same as the men's, a very dangerous admission in a context where any difference looks like inferiority.

Take, for example, the biological differences between women

and men—not just size and strength, but also body shape, muscle fatigue processes, pain experience and expression, hormonal differences that may affect our reactions to toxic chemicals, menstrual cramps that may become disabling under some workplace conditions, pregnancy that may keep us from doing some tasks, nursing babies who may be affected by chemicals. When women's biology is ignored, working women suffer, have more work accidents, and have more musculoskeletal problems than men. Right now, women hesitate to mention any differences because of the danger that those differences will be invoked to deny them access to jobs and promotions. And that danger is real. But in my view, our silence is hurting women economically and making us ill.

Why should we try to deny differences instead of insisting on adapting and redesigning equipment, workspaces, and training? Yes, men arrived in many workplaces well before women, so it is understandable that jobs were designed as a function of how most cis men's bodies worked. But if women's bodies are not to be treated as second-class, we need to consider what concrete changes are necessary. Otherwise, women entering non-traditional jobs with physical requirements will continue to be at extra risk for accidents and illnesses.

My government has been complicit in this attempt to deny women's experience with aggressive colleagues and passive employers, but denial has not worked. As of 2018, fifteen years after the first affirmative action program, women in Quebec were fewer than 2 percent of all construction workers.

This is why a first step toward reconciling equality with women's health and safety has to be to get rid of the shame that overcomes us when we are attacked or ignored in the workplace. I know that shame well. I remember the first time I sat down with nine other professors during the mid-1970s to decide how to improve our cell biology BSc program. I was the only woman in the room and the only (at that time) molecular geneticist in the university, and I had just gotten a big research grant. The group decided to rewrite the biology program to take into account the emerging knowledge about genes and cell biology, and they looked around for someone to take on the responsibility. They suggested Jean-Pierre, then Robert, then Charles, then Marc, none of whom had any particular qualifications. I remember looking down at my arms and touching myself to make sure I really existed in the room, in flesh and blood. But I didn't say anything, convinced that the men had noticed some fatal disqualification I hadn't realized I had. And I stayed silent for years.

I know now that we need to combat our shame and fear head-on. In particular, we need to document the invisible risks in our work and direct attention to them, while recognizing that the jobs men do have their own specific types of risks. And we need to develop ways to work together, in solidarity, to protect each other while working toward those goals.

During the 1980s, Donna Mergler and I began collaborating with a lively group of researchers to form what eventually became the CINBIOSE research centre in environmental and occupational health (Centre de recherche interdisciplinaire sur le bien-être, la santé, la société et l'environnement).[12] In 1993 the occupational health scientists formed a partnership with the women's committees and health and safety committees of Quebec's three major trade unions, aiming to improve women's health and safety at work. Over the following seventeen years, the ergonomists led interventions in over twenty workplaces, and the legal experts produced important public policy innovations as well as advice on collective agreements and workplace practices.[13] A younger group of researchers is now leading these efforts, and we are trying to make sense of what we did.

The next chapters will explain our approach and present some of our interventions and what happened to them.

2.
SHAME AND SILENCE IN HEALTH CARE

Lucie Dagenais is a classic "union maid," devoted to improving working conditions. She was trained as a nurse and played an important role in founding nurses' unions and in maintaining Quebec's public health system.[1] Her union sent her to headquarters to work at the education and training service of the Confédération des syndicats nationaux (CSN). She is very smart, and always hoping for new ideas that will help workers.

When I got back from Paris and my ergonomics course in 1991, Lucie put me to work right away, training hospital workers on how to protect their bodies from overuse and injury.[2] Since hospital workers are surrounded by health professionals, they had already heard over and over that they should bend at the knee and not at the waist when lifting patients, and that they should pay attention to the signs on the patients' doors, warning of infections, radiation, and chemicals. But learning a set of rules didn't give them more time or space to do the job safely.[3] The personal support worker (PSW) job, most often (80 percent) held by women, still counts among those most likely to cause work accidents, particularly among older women.[4] In Quebec, six of every hundred full-time PSWs are compensated for work-related musculoskeletal problems every year, more than any other type of hospital worker in patient care.[5] In Ontario, a 2019 union report describes a "staffing crisis" affecting these workers, arising from job cuts but also difficulties in recruitment due to low pay, overwork, lack of respect, and poor conditions generally.[6] In Quebec, during the COVID-19 pandemic, understaffing became critical, resulting in a desperate shuffling of workers among shifts, departments, and hospitals that infected workers and patients alike.

When I started talking with the PSWs about how to analyze their work, I learned that their job was also a battleground for employment equity. Before the 1960s, female and male PSWs occupied explicitly sex-identified job titles like "nursing assistant (female)" and "stretcher-bearer (male)," and the men were paid more. When explicit sex distinctions became illegal, the jobs were renamed "light work (LW)" and "heavy work (HW)," with higher pay for HW. LW, almost always assigned to women, included direct patient care such as dressing, washing, and feeding patients, while HW, almost always done by men, involved restraining aggressive patients, lifting patients, or transferring them from wheelchairs into beds.

Because of legal and union pressures for equity in employment, the LW and HW job titles were merged in the 1979–82 CSN collective agreement. But ten years later, there was no consensus that this had been a good thing. In our training sessions, both women and men said the merger had been a mistake, that women were not strong enough to move patients. Everyone agreed that women PSWs in the merged job titles were injuring themselves and men were being overworked, doing extra lifting to compensate for their weaker colleagues. And in fact, women in this job had a third more recognized occupational accidents compared to men.[7]

According to the PSWs, some hospital departments had tried to ensure that at least one man would be hired on each floor to do the heavy lifting, but tribunals found that this practice discriminated against women, so where it persisted, it was hidden. Subsequent jurisprudence reinforced identical requirements for women and men in this job. Nevertheless, women and men agreed that the nurses would always ask men, never women, to help them with physically demanding tasks. Everyone complained that the extra work was unfair to the men. Older men especially expressed fear of back problems from the extra lifting.[8] I thought I had come across an interesting case of discrimination against men.

After our sessions, we discussed with the union women's committee how the work of PSWs could be made better for women and men. Coincidentally, an occupational health physician contacted us because she was concerned that the job merger had been harmful to the PSWs' health, with both women and men working beyond their strength. With her support, we were able to get a Canadian government grant to study the situation.

We then visited management and union executives at fifteen hospitals in different regions of Quebec to get an overview of how the job title merger had gone and get a sense of their willingness to participate in an ergonomic analysis. These official respondents were unanimous in saying that the jobs had been successfully merged and that women and men did exactly the same tasks. However, all but two hospitals refused to take part in our study, saying "Ne réveillons pas le chat qui dort" (Let sleeping dogs lie). When pushed, both unions and management explained that the merger had been painful and controversial, and that they were afraid to reopen old wounds and poison relations between female and male PSWs. Women and men had often been opposed, and also divided among themselves over the merger. We could see that it was not going to be easy to discuss gendered job assignments.

Observing gendered work

Two hospitals finally accepted our study, on the explicit condition that our report would focus on reducing work-related injuries rather than on gender. PSWs in a third hospital recruited by Julie Dussault, a master's level student, helped us by responding to a short questionnaire listing the various physical components of their work; they rated the difficulty of each operation (turn patient in bed, make a bed . . .). Given what I had heard already, I wasn't surprised that women respondents rated all operations as significantly more physically demanding, on average, than did men.

With another ergonomist, Diane Elabidi, I interviewed women and men and observed work for a hundred hours in four departments employing a 60 percent female workforce. We chose the people to observe so as to get a sample of different times of day, patient types (dementia vs. others), and genders. We only observed workers with some experience.

The work was indeed very physical. We saw the PSWs move patients around in bed to wash and dress them, talking to them all the while. They pushed, pulled, and lifted patients from beds into and out of wheelchairs and stretchers. Depending on the needs of the patients, they gave them showers, fed them, and moved them from place to place. They dealt with physical resistance and even violence from patients and occasional criticism from patients' families. The job could be taxing—we saw a PSW give a shower to Lily, a woman with dementia—a long, complicated, and challenging procedure where she transferred the woman from her wheelchair to a sling arrangement in a shower, then washed her and transferred her back—only to have the woman defecate in the chair and on herself before her diaper could be reinstalled. "Oh, Lily," the PSW sighed, before restarting the shower procedure.

We constructed an observation grid for operations in the two hospitals. All observed operations were classed as "very physically demanding," "physically demanding," or "not demanding," based on the average of the workers' answers to the questionnaire (not distinguished by gender). For each physically demanding operation, we noted whether it was shared with a colleague and the gender of the observed worker and (where applicable) the colleague.

The results astonished us. The data were entirely opposite to what we had heard. When we analyzed our observations, there was no sign that men were doing the lion's share of physically demanding operations, and they were certainly not helping nurses more than the women. Yes, all PSWs shared a great deal of the physical demands of their work, as hospital guidelines suggested: 45 percent of all physical operations and 62 percent of the more demanding operations were done in pairs. But we found that the women performed 30 percent more physical tasks per hour (15 percent more demanding tasks per hour) compared to men, and that women performed them alone about as often as did men.[9] More of women's time was spent in direct care with patients. Most unexpectedly, nurses were *four times more* likely to ask for help with physical tasks from female PSWs than from males, while male PSWs were significantly *more* likely than females to ask for help from a nurse. Occasionally—three times during the hundred hours of observations—we did observe that a male PSW was asked to perform a particularly dangerous task explicitly because of his sex: twice men were called to lift or move morbidly obese patients and once to restrain an aggressive patient. One of the men refused to lift a heavy patient alone, insisting on help from the female PSWs present who were hanging back. We did not observe any similar physical demands placed on women explicitly because of their gender.

Presenting the results

We had a meeting with all the PSWs in one department to get feed-back on these results. I have to admit that we didn't even think of concealing the striking results about gender, despite our promise to the hospital authorities. We did want to suggest several ways the employer could diminish physical demands. But we didn't get far enough to discuss solutions. Vincent, the union president, said straight out that he didn't believe our results. No matter what our numbers said, he knew that women were doing less of the physical work. He told us, in her presence, that Rose refused to lift heavy loads, citing the fact that she was a middle-aged woman as her reason for refusing. (We had not observed Rose at work.) He said that if he looked at the schedule and saw he was to work with Rose on a certain day, he knew it would be a bad day for him. Rose was not ashamed of this; she said right out that she didn't think women should do lifting and she had been happier before the jobs were merged.

To examine Vincent's perception, I asked all those present to fill out a piece of paper with the names of everyone else in the department and write down (confidentially) if it was a good day or a bad day when they had to work with them. The lists for bad days contained two names: Rose was on everyone's list, but so was Jacob, who was not at the meeting. Vincent told us that it would be a bad day if he had to work with Jacob because Jacob was lazy, but that he felt that Rose's behaviour meant "women" weren't able to do the work. He complained that some newly hired women (whom we had not observed because we only included experienced workers) were "toothpicks," too slightly built to do the job.

I could understand Rose's point of view, since I was her age (fifties) and would have had trouble with all the lifting, but I resented her for putting the other women in a bad position. I was also annoyed that Jacob's behaviour didn't seem to affect anyone's opinion of young men, but then, unlike Rose, Jacob had never explicitly pinpointed his gender by saying, "I'm lazy because I'm a young man."

We presented our results, separately, to workers and supervisors. The exchanges with workers, held in gender-mixed groups, became somewhat acrimonious and uncomfortable, with both men and women disputing our results on the frequency of physically demanding tasks done by women. Nevertheless, some women later told us privately that they believed our data. Two (female) supervisors also said that our report squared with their observations and that the women were working very hard. But the local union (Vincent was its president) showed no interest in the results. I was struck by the silence of the women, and stymied about how to go further with the study.

Gender is easily forgotten

We produced a report to the hospitals and unions with suggestions on how to reduce the physical demands of work, by supporting teamwork and making lifting equipment more available. We also noted that gender stereotypes seemed to present a danger for musculoskeletal problems and work accidents for both women and men: women seemed to be overworking because they were accused of not doing their share, and men were being asked to do some extreme tasks because of their gender. Our report was vetted and endorsed by two other ergonomists, Dominic and Helen, who had previously studied the PSWs' job.

Six months after our final report on the PSWs, I happened to cross Dominic's path. I mentioned that I had just published a book on women's occupational health and safety, *One-Eyed Science* (1998),[10] and he replied, "Why a book on women? Men's jobs, women's jobs, there's no difference. A woman PSW, a man PSW, it's the same job." I reminded him that the report he'd examined and approved had said exactly the opposite, but he seemed not to remember.

I had trouble understanding how Dominic could have so quickly forgotten our research results, but I realized that, in his daily work in hospitals, he was never asked to think about gender. He had to make suggestions to improve work for everyone, and our report had indicated several possibilities, so he concentrated on those. The specific occupational health and safety problem that consisted of women overworking because they were afraid of being considered a burden was not a visible ergonomics problem and he would never be asked to deal with it, given the hospitals' reluctance to even mention gender and the women's shamed silence. Was Dominic, a soft-spoken, friendly guy, reluctant to stir the hornet's nest of workplace gender relations? Was he just as glad to forget about pesky social problems and stick to his own area of competence? Not impossible.

When we examined the scientific literature, however, we found that we were not the first to describe male-female differences in PSWs' work activity. In 1987, Monique Lortie had also found that male PSWs did fewer physically demanding operations than women, and the differences she found were even more striking.[11] She explained why women did more of the demanding operations by her observation that women often divided one difficult patient-handling operation into several, somewhat easier parts. The women had discovered specific techniques that made patient handling easier for smaller people, like using mattress pads to slide patients around on their beds, rather than picking them up bodily and moving them. These differences in technique could have applied to our data as well, but they did not explain why nurses preferentially asked women for help. Because nurses were members of a rival, hostile union, we had no access to their collective interpretation of our results, but nursing managers told us their impression was that conscientious nurses were trying to avoid being accused of exploiting the male PSWs.

I should emphasize that our results concerned only two hospitals, and that we were only allowed to present the results in one of the two. Union-management relationships were not particularly harmonious, and management, who had not been enthusiastic at the outset, showed no interest in going further with the study or even with the proposals for change in the job environment that did not involve gender. The local hospital's union was not pushing for change either, since they said they didn't believe our results.

It was surprising that managers did not seem to feel that they had to do anything about the situation, even though they were conscious of the male-female tensions. They seemed to have no idea how to intervene, and only expressed interest in not reopening the wounds incurred at the time of the job merger. We couldn't attribute their cold feet just to the fact that Vincent was the union president and could make trouble; the other participating hospital also ignored the study results and the first thirteen hospitals we'd approached had refused to participate.

Julie Dussault, who had contacted the third hospital independently, presented her results there without referring to gender, making interesting suggestions for how the work should be organized. For instance, she said that the practice of assigning each PSW to a separate group of two-patient rooms should be changed. When one PSW was assigned to both patients in a room, she would have to leave the room to ask for help. But if two PSWs were assigned jointly to sets of rooms, they would automatically help each other with pushing, pulling, and lifting. Julie's suggestions were adopted in that hospital and pleased everyone. So, when gender was not mentioned, our suggestions could lead to change.

Shame and taboo

Looking back on our experiences, how can I explain the difficulty we faced when we tried to get both workers and colleagues to accept the results? This is really a story about the power of shame and denial. Think about all those women feeling ashamed because they were doing less than the men, and feeling compelled to hurt their backs to make up for it. And all those observers forgetting their observations.

I have to admit that my posture as a neutral ergonomist working to answer union requests didn't help. I was feeling ashamed myself—first for having accepted the condition of silence about gender, and then for transgressing it. Although I was straightforward in saying to Vincent that I thought he was being unfair, I didn't do what I probably should have done—call a meeting with just the women and maybe even the (all-female) supervisors. On the other hand, it wouldn't have helped if everyone started saying it was the men who weren't doing their share; in fact, both men and women were overworked in this time of job cuts and subcontracting, and the men were being preferentially called on in the more extreme and dangerous (though rarer) situations.

I am struck by the fact that Julie was able to make more positive change by never mentioning gender. We have seen this several times since. My colleague Nicole Vézina and her students have succeeded in helping a lot of women without specifically mentioning gender (see chapter 6). I don't want to make it sound easier than it is, but they have identified and improved a number of industrial jobs where women are confined to doing a series of incredibly fast manipulations on a product handed to them by men in a preceding job position. For example, one of Nicole's students, Idil Suge, observed a kitchen job where a woman had to sort dishes put on a conveyor belt by two men. She had to separate plates, glasses, and cups of different sizes and put them in different places while inspecting them for quality. Her output was therefore at least twice that of each of the men, but no one had noticed. She became exhausted and her arms and shoulders hurt. Without mentioning gender, Suge succeeded in getting an assistant for the woman worker. Problem solved.

Puzzles for feminists

So should we just shut up about gender? Is it a good idea to do reforms on one job at a time without going into the wider context? But then, was the woman in the dish-sorting job left feeling ashamed that she needed a helper? Did she feel guilty for complaining? Why did she have to wait so long for change? And especially, was management going to make the same mistake again?

What does all this tell us about biological differences? Is Rose typical of aging women in health care? Are the male-female strength difference and the extra pain women suffer important enough that we should go back to explicitly gender-segregated job titles? Should Rose have been given modified work, so that she would not have had to use her gender as the pretext for making her colleagues help her? It is important to remember that some of the aging men also said they needed modified work.

And what the heck can we do with Dominic, the ergonomist who forgot the research results he had signed off on less than a year earlier? Tell him to look at gender and hope we haven't encouraged stereotyping? Or be happy he is gender-blind and be grateful for all the positive changes he has made in women's work in hospitals?

Throughout this study and during several others, I wondered why we had so much trouble making changes. But more explicitly feminist interventions didn't necessarily help, as we were to find out when we studied another case of job desegregation, this time in cleaning.

3.
A FEMINIST INTERVENTION THAT HURT WOMEN?

Quebec hospitals are publicly owned, and hospital cleaners are government employees, unionized and relatively well-paid as cleaners' pay goes. During the 1990s, the province was trying to save money, and cleaning, the least prestigious of hospital jobs, seemed like a good place to cut. It didn't look to politicians or the public like cleaning had anything to do with the hospitals' "central mission" of curing the sick. (Just as during the COVID-19 pandemic, there was strong public sympathy for doctors, nurses, and PSWs, but cleaners' exposure to infection was hardly ever mentioned.) Hospital administrations shared the public's low opinion of cleaning and they cut expenses, reducing the number of cleaners, contracting out the cleaning jobs, and enlarging the number of floors assigned per cleaner.[1]

But the unions were convinced that cleaning was vital to patient care because good hygiene prevented disease from spreading. They started a campaign against outsourcing and job intensification. As part of the campaign, they used the UQAM-union agreement to access our services, since our team had studied this job. We were to teach about biological and ergonomic risks, such as exposure to germs, corrosive chemicals, and awkward postures. The workers wanted to know how to protect themselves and what equipment and environmental changes to ask for.

But during the training sessions, cleaners also complained bitterly about their terrible communication with nursing staff, which made it hard for the cleaners to organize their work and protect their health. Cleaning was at the bottom of the hospital hierarchy, so I also heard a lot about how cleaners and even cleaning managers were excluded from decision-making. They were never part of consultations on equipment purchases, room design, and furniture choices, despite their effects on the ease, or not, of cleaning. Cleaners also shocked me with reports of insults from the families of hospital patients and other people who had no idea of how little power the cleaners had over the level of dirt in the hospital.

Cleaning, like health care, had initially been segregated by gender. Women working in hospitals had traditionally been assigned to "cleaning (women)." They dusted furniture, cleaned toilets, and emptied wastebaskets. Men were assigned to "cleaning (men)" and mopped, polished floors, and pushed vacuum cleaners. They got paid more than the women. In the 1960s, the job titles were changed respectively to "cleaning (light work)" and "cleaning (heavy work)" with little change in job content. The HW jobs were still done almost exclusively by men and received higher pay than the LW jobs done mostly by women and occasionally by injured, ill, or aging men.

During the 1970s and 80s, the union had tried to diminish the female-male wage gap in hospital cleaning by raising wages in women's jobs. The women's committees had to battle not only the hospitals and the government, but also the many male cleaners who maintained that the women's jobs were easier. It was a long struggle, but the pay differential was abolished in the 1980s. The separate job titles persisted, however. I should note that this is only one of many situations in Quebec, North America, and Europe, where tasks assigned to "cleaners" (women) are different from those of "janitors," "custodians," or "maintenance workers," almost always done by men.

In the 1990s training sessions, cleaners voiced their health concerns. They were not allowed to access any information on patient diagnoses, so they didn't know which patients were contagious. They were quite scared when they went into patients' rooms, especially when they saw nurses and doctors taking special precautions. Some of them managed their fear by using their cleaning chemicals undiluted, exposing themselves to potential toxic effects. They explained not using the recommended dilutions by the fact that their cleaning territory had been expanded and they wanted to be sure to kill all the germs in the little time they had available. Besieged by exhausted and angry cleaners, the union needed to know more about their problems. The women's committee of the union was especially concerned because cleaning operations were segregated by gender and the women's jobs were hit harder by the job cuts.

In contacting us, the union women's committee and health and safety reps wanted to know what job hazards there were and how they were distributed by gender. They wanted evidence to combat the job cuts. The cleaners were happy to collaborate and got North Hospital to allow us to observe work there.[2]

The ergonomic intervention

We started our study in 1994. The only source of funds for ergonomics (work analysis) research was then in social sciences, so we oriented our grant application toward questions of gender and sex and their influence on the division of assigned tasks and actual work activity.[3] We got enough money to hire two graduate students,

Céline Chatigny and Julie Courville, to distribute a short question-naire about physical symptoms.[4] We observed the cleaners' work for 60.25 hours (25.5 hours for light work and 34.75 hours for heavy work) spread out over a period of weeks, during day and evening shifts.[5]

After an initial round of observations, I asked Céline and Julie to describe the work and give me their first impressions. Since they were both feminists, I was concerned that they not allow their own views on gender—or mine—to bias their observations. I wanted to develop an observation grid quickly, since I hoped a grid would allow them to check categories of movements and actions as objec-tively as possible, without thinking too much about the gender of the workers. I need not have worried. When we met to debrief, I was at the same time reassured and quite surprised to find that Céline and Julie had forgotten about gender. Their experiences observing the work had focused their attention on understanding and improv-ing the organizational and material conditions of all cleaners. And in talking with them and, later, in watching the cleaners, I too for-got about gender, distracted by all the obstacles to cleaning: what happened when a low-prestige, invisible male cleaner tried to mop a corridor filled with wheelchairs, drug carts, and high-prestige doctors on very important business; how many pictures of the grandchildren, boxes of candy, and magazines the female cleaners had to move in order to dust the bedside tables. We had plenty of data on women and men; we just forgot to think about gender, just as Dominic had done with the study of health care aides.

It is also true that workers and managers in general say they find it strange to discuss gender in relation to their work. But our forgetfulness during this study was especially bizarre in light of our major finding about the cleaners. When we analyzed our notes and grids, we saw not only a strict division of assigned tasks by job title, but also added, unassigned tasks associated with workers' gender.

Each office, hospital room, and common area was cleaned twice: once by a man assigned to "heavy work" and once by a woman assigned to "light work"; they worked in teams. Most time in HW was spent mopping and vacuuming floors, washing large surfaces, and doing any work requiring use of a ladder. In some hospitals, workers had been told, erroneously, that it was illegal for a woman to use a ladder or that insurance wouldn't cover costs if a woman had an accident on a ladder. So any time nurses would have needed to climb, they called a male cleaner—to change a light bulb, to clean a vent, to close a reluctant curtain. Male cleaners assigned to HW said nurses asked them to do many tasks perceived as male, from pushing heavy objects to calming and even restraining obstreperous psychiatric patients. Similar gender differences in cleaners' tasks have also been described in the United States.[6]

"Light work," on the other hand, consisted of cleaning and dusting small objects and anything that could be reached from a standing, kneeling, or stretching position, such as bedside tables, chairs, bedsteads, curtain rods, medical equipment, and toilets. LW cleaners were also responsible for waste disposal, emptying over 150 garbage bins per day. To prevent contamination, they had to change the plastic bin liners every time. Although the bins could be big, small, or medium, there was only one size of bin liner. When the liner was too small for the size of the bin, the LW cleaners had to shake it out and tie a knot in it to keep it from falling to the bottom of the bin, where waste would accumulate around it and soil the bin. When the liner was too big, the cleaners had, again, to shake it out and tie a knot in it to keep it snug around the top of the bin. At the end of the day, the LW cleaners' wrists were sore from all the knot tying and from shaking out the bags. The knot tying was not listed on the inventories of tasks that consultants had used to plan staffing, but it was an important, invisible, health-damaging part of the women's jobs.

According to Julie and Céline, LW tasks in general were more often omitted from the official lists of tasks, so that LW was understaffed and cleaners were forced to hurry to finish their assigned tasks. Equipment forgotten in rooms and never used or inventoried still had to be cleaned, patients' personal belongings had to be moved in order to dust their tables, and so on.

Gender stereotypes also resulted in conflicts over work assignments. Was it acceptable for a woman cleaning a bathroom mirror (LW) to use a ladder (HW), or should she wobble dangerously on the edge of the sink or toilet? Should HW or LW (or nurses) clean up when a nurse spilled urine, given that urine is associated with waste and toilets (LW) but also with floor cleaning (HW)?

When we started to look at the effects of task segregation on workers' health, we found that the male-female division of tasks corresponded to a difference in physical work activity. The postures of those doing LW were more varied and involved more extreme contortions than in HW. LW cleaners stooped, stretched, and bent over more often, while those in HW stood upright, walked, and pushed mops and polishers. Timed movements were faster in LW than in HW, but movement amplitude was smaller because dusting bedside tables and furniture requires finer movements than mopping floors. Surprisingly, though, there was some overlap in the weights manipulated: although, on the average, HW manipulated heavier weights, some full wastebaskets lifted by LW were heavier than almost anything lifted by HW.

We next found that the division of work activity corresponded to a gender difference in reported pain and fatigue, although both women and men were likely to suffer pain associated with their cleaning work. Nineteen workers (nine female, ten male) filled out a short questionnaire; the women reported significantly more neck/shoulder fatigue but less back fatigue than the men. This was not surprising, since neck and shoulder symptoms can be associated with cramped postures and intense hand/arm movements, while back fatigue can be associated with lifting heavy weights.

Our major conclusion was that the managers and consultants had underestimated the physical challenges of LW. With the workers' help, we put in a report with eighty-four proposals for change in equipment, procedures, and installations. We suggested that management think about desegregating cleaning tasks, although we weren't sure whether to recommend desegregation. A friendly young human resources manager at North Hospital put many of our proposals into effect. He bought different-sized bin liners, held meetings to build dialogue between nurses and cleaners, and corrected the inventory of tasks. We left the hospital satisfied with our work and wrote our scientific articles.[7]

Changes, 1995–2007

Over the following twelve years, cleaning work in hospitals changed considerably. First, epidemics of contagious illnesses like *Clostridium difficile* broke out in many hospitals, leading to concern with hygiene and slowing the trend to cutting and outsourcing cleaners' jobs. Second, a government pay equity examination raised the pay for LW so that their pay became higher than for HW; the commission had been influenced by our report on the job content of LW, among other evidence. Third, several hospitals merged the HW and LW job titles, sometimes citing our report where we had mentioned that each space was cleaned once by HW and once by LW. Where they were merged, the new job was called "heavy work." Therefore, although the number of LW employees dropped precipitously over this period, the number of employees designated HW, now male and female, stayed constant. We were quite proud that our research had led directly to job improvement in North Hospital and indirectly to what looked like a better deal for women workers in hospital cleaning.

In 2007, nine years after the end of the first study, the union women's committee asked us to look at the cleaning job again. They wanted to know whether to support the trend to merging LW and HW into a job with combined tasks.

In a hospital we had not studied, Central Hospital, unionized women were blocking the merger, saying they didn't want to do certain tasks in HW and that they feared being forced to leave if the jobs were merged. They pointed out that, because of the pay equity success, the LW jobs being cut paid more than the HW jobs they would be taking. This was happening because the pay equity committee was set up to compare women's jobs not with the men working alongside them, but with a majority-male job doing work similar to the women's. The aim had been to improve equity between women and men workers generally, not among cleaners. Since the HW cleaners were assigned to different tasks from the LW cleaners, LW was compared, instead, to similar types of cleaning jobs usually done by men, such as cleaning animal cages. The committee never examined the salary of HW, since its mandate included only pay equity for women's jobs.

The pay equity committee had thus raised the LW salary to the level of the comparable male groups, who actually earned more than HW hospital cleaners. The women did not want to lose this advantage by being merged with HW. Although they would not suffer an immediate loss of pay, they were afraid for their future salary increases and scared by the potentially "heavy" job demands.

But we couldn't study their work, because Central Hospital refused access for our study. So we examined two hospitals where HW and LW had already been merged: the original hospital (North Hospital) and another one (South Hospital). We were especially curious to see what had happened to the work in North Hospital in the years since our last visit.

Our professional and feminist pride took quite a beating. We found that the number and proportion of women cleaners had dropped sharply since our original study of North Hospital, from 37 percent to 23 percent.[8] Many of the older women had left. The women in the merged LW-HW job were much less senior than in 1994–95, and significantly younger than the men.

We again observed the work and interviewed the cleaners. We saw that the work activity of women and men in the merged job title still differed, with men spending twice as much time on mopping as women, and women spending twice as much time cleaning toilets as men. In interviews, we were told that some men objected on principle to cleaning toilets, saying, "I don't clean toilets at home, why would I do it here?"[9]

A close examination of tasks in both North and South Hospitals showed that some assignments were unpopular with most women and many men. One example was trash compacting in South Hospital, which involved exceptionally heavy loads as well as general stinkiness. One barrier for women entering the merged job was that trash compacting was perceived as impossible for women. In 2012, a student, Bénédicte Calvet, examined this job more closely with a view to making it less dangerous and unpleasant. She documented many difficulties for smaller, less muscular people and made a lot of suggestions, but management neither paid for this study nor committed to any changes. Given all the ongoing budget cuts in the health care sector, the local union's priority was fighting work intensification rather than facilitating entry for women.

A terrifying finding during our follow-up was that women's rate of occupational accidents had climbed to be much higher than men's, as often happens when women enter men's jobs without any changes in training, equipment, or tools (see chapter 1). Pain reports had also changed: men still had a bit more back pain, and women, a bit more arm pain, but there were no longer statistically significant male-female differences. All workers, especially men, reported more fatigue in their legs than before; this might have been related to the intervening job cuts that had enlarged the areas to be cleaned. Sadly, only about a third of the environmental changes we'd recommended had persisted over the intervening twelve years. The nice young man in human resources was long gone, the union executive had changed, the garbage bin liners were back to their old, single size, and the cleaners and nurses were still arguing over who would do what. No one remembered what had happened to the changes.

What happened?

Why were there fewer women in cleaning and why were they having more accidents? There were many reasons, some due to gender (social roles), some to sex (biological differences), and some to local dynamics in these workplaces.

Women at North Hospital who had been doing "light work" for a long time told us that they were unable to do "heavy work." We had no direct contact with those who had left after the job titles merged, but their colleagues told us that the older women had reacted like those at Central Hospital, objecting to the merger and then taking early retirement. Among the women we had talked to in 1994, no one had questioned the gender stereotyping in their task assignments. The LW women had enjoyed being paired with a man to clean the offices. Aside from everything else, it was fun to have someone to talk to. One married couple had arranged to be paired and enjoyed the time together at work. So if we listened to the women, we heard no reason why they would have wanted the jobs to merge.

What if we listened to the employer? In our first study of light and heavy work, managers had justified the job segregation by stereotyping; they described women as more meticulous and conscientious cleaners than men, whereas men were stronger but more careless. If you wanted someone to clean the big bosses' offices, it should be a women "because they dust even behind the books." However, this supposed aptitude for careful cleaning did not appear to weigh heavily in hiring after the merger, compared to the fact that men were perceived as better able to handle machines and lift weights.

By 2007–2008, managers (all male) gave at least lip service to the idea that the women and men who worked for them had equal capacities to clean, although the South Hospital managers worried about finding women who could be assigned to the trash compactor. They said they made no distinction between male and female applicants (it would have been illegal to do so) but that women appeared to be reluctant to apply for "heavy" cleaning jobs. They didn't mention making any special effort to recruit women or even wanting more women to apply. Maybe dusting behind the books wasn't that important.

Feminist yearnings were nowhere to be found among the workers, either, although when pressed, the women who had accepted the HW classification said there was no difference between women and men and that desegregation had been a good thing. Like the communications technicians in chapter 1, the women doing HW also appeared afraid to seem different from the men and far from able to ask for any adaptation in tools, equipment, or training. None of them protested about doing the extra toilets, even though that task required many awkward postures and contortions.

Was it a mistake to merge the jobs?

Our experiences made us wonder whether desegregation of manual jobs is a bad idea. Certainly, none of the women cleaners had been pushing for it, and none of those we interviewed mentioned any concrete way their work had improved. No one, female or male, even said they liked the fact that the tasks were less repetitive.

The employers, on the other hand, were happy with the situation. They appeared to have merged the job titles for two reasons, both of which involved cost reductions. First, once pay equity was established at the provincial level, the "light work" designation became more expensive than "heavy work." Doing away with LW altogether saved money. Second, a job merger saved time because each space was now cleaned by only one person, in theory saving time and therefore money. A bonus: the merger could easily be justified on the grounds of gender equality; the union could not object to it, especially since gender equality in task assignments and remuneration had been a union demand for years. Downward pressure on costs coming from the government meant, however, that there was no money to spend on environmental and organizational improvements that would make tasks easier for smaller people—or indeed for anyone. On the contrary, increasing time pressure was making the job more difficult, driving out those who had the most trouble doing it. Many of those who left were older women who had spent years successfully coping with a traditionally gendered set of tasks and had not asked for the change. So both groups of women hospital workers had lost out when their jobs were merged. The women PSWs (chapter 2) were doing more lifting, and the women cleaners were having more accidents.

We saw no pressure from workers or their local unions to adapt the job to women workers, possibly because they were afraid to sound as if they were saying their female members were weak. The national women's committee of the union, on the other hand, was interested in pursuing the issue of job desegregation. It published a pamphlet on relationships between women and men at work, presenting several of our interventions in hospitals and other workplaces.[10] The pamphlet, beautifully written with lots of examples, was meant to be a basis for discussions in joint meetings of local health and safety committees (mostly men) and status of women committees (all female). Unfortunately, the first joint meeting was a disaster. The discussion got out of hand, with some people taking an accusatory tone, others going on at length about their personal situations, and others reduced to silence. Some men felt unfairly accused and some women felt intimidated. The experiment was not repeated, despite the fact that the status of women committees in this union confederation have traditionally been very strong and active.

Still, interviewed years later by independent researchers, the feminists in both committees were happy with our efforts and delighted that the segregated jobs had been successfully merged.

Puzzles for feminists

Although our studies had probably resulted in higher pay for a number of women during a short period, they had not done away with the gender segregation of tasks nor had they made jobs more available to women. On the contrary. We had to wonder what to say to the women in Central Hospital who were asking me and the union health and safety people to say straight out that women were biologically unable to do "heavy work" and that job segregation at their hospital should be maintained. And as feminists, we couldn't ignore the fact that no women actually working in LW had put in any request to integrate LW and HW. More recognition and money for the physical challenges in LW, yes. Doing HW tasks, no. Had the women been induced to accept what turned out to be a short-term economic gain, only to be faced with deteriorating working conditions? Our experiences with both groups of hospital workers left us with two questions.

First, is job segregation in jobs with a physical component a good thing for women?

Would it have been better for all the women to have kept the old job segregation? Had those who left when the jobs were merged felt inadequate? Or were they just protecting their health? Did they feel that they were unqualified to do "heavy work"? Was it a bad thing for women in a women-identified profession (LW) to lose their specific place in hospital work? Did women in the merged job feel ashamed of being different from their male colleagues? Were some men ashamed of profiting from their physical advantages?

Although a strong unspoken current of sexism and anti-women bias underlay all of what we saw and heard in this workplace, we saw no way to get a handle on it, nor did the union women's committee that had sent us there.

And what about the managers during all this? We saw no evidence that they had been proactive either at the time of the merger or after. No one in management had noticed that women's accident rate was higher than men's, and we felt bad for mentioning it, since no prevention activities were going to be initiated and the only possible consequence was more prejudice against women.

I believe that these debates are hampered not only by taboos, but also by the many unknowns and even more numerous myths about women's and men's bodies. I will consider this question from a scientific point of view in the next two chapters. After that I will confront my own demons. I would like to know what we could have done differently—our second question.

Second, could we have helped women more?

Do these experiences offer any hints for feminist interventions in workplaces? How should we intervene to improve women's work? Is there any way the women in the workplace can be more involved in guiding the research process, given their limited availability and the unions' tiny budgets for freeing up time for discussions? I will discuss gender and ergonomic intervention in chapters 6, 7, and 8.

PART II.
SEGREGATED
BODIES

4.
JOBS AND BODIES

A s usual, it was a student who called my attention to something important. Micheline Boucher, a graduate student in ergonomics, was studying an attempt to desegregate jobs that had run into roadblocks. Three years after a city had been ordered to hire more women, only 22 of its 201 job titles had any women at all. The union women's committee asked us to find out what was happening. Among the jobs, gardening had the most women, so we decided to study that job. Micheline observed the gardeners' work and interviewed 57 of them, all 30 women and the 27 men hired at about the same time. At the end of one day watching gardeners, she came bounding into my office. "They don't do the same things!" she exclaimed. She had found that in about half of work teams, women were assigned specific tasks. They would plant small plants and uproot weeds, while the men would plant big plants and bushes and operate lawnmowers.[1] It had kind of evolved that way. Although, theoretically, the women had entered the exact same jobs as the men, a gendered subdivision of labour had quickly been established.

We could imagine that this kind of stereotypical redivision

of physical labour by sex could have been be a reaction to the court-ordered job desegregation. The men or the supervisors could have been resisting women's "invasion." But that city was not alone. Twenty-five years later, when I was on a bicycle trip in Vietnam, I passed by some municipal landscapers in Ho Chi Minh City. As in Quebec, the women were all crouching down and weeding, and the men were standing up and hoeing.

We have observed gender differences in physical task assignments even in jobs where women are in the majority. According to the most recent data from Statistics Canada, food service is the fourteenth-most-common women's job, and 79 percent of food servers in Canada are women.[2] Their union asked us to study their job because they were tired of being insulted and looked down on. "Tell them we're intelligent!" they said. Eve Laperrière, a PhD student, was interested in the project since she had worked in restaurants to support herself through university. She deftly negotiated her way into a restaurant chain so she could observe the work, and developed a questionnaire that sixty-four servers answered online.[3]

The restaurants were smallish and priced toward the low end. Servers were on their feet and moving all the time. They carried heavy plates and glasses back and forth from kitchen to table to kitchen. They got tired quickly. There was no place for them to sit, even on their breaks, because management thought it would irritate customers to see the servers sitting while they were waiting hungrily for their meal.

Servers really did have to be intelligent—they had to think and plan a lot. They had to figure out what customers wanted, remember it, describe it to the kitchen staff, watch for the dishes they had ordered, deliver them and any side dishes to the right people at the right tables, and take care of billing and payment. They had to be alert for the patron who wanted another glass of water or the one who changed her mind about having her hamburger well done.

At the same time, they had to make sure the coffee machine was working, water glasses were full, and salt and pepper shakers were functional.

> "In my mind, I'm repeating: water glass / bill / ketchup / coffee-tea / water glass / bill / ketchup / coffee-tea . . ." (a female food server)[4]

They had to watch the customers carefully—are they signalling, are they upset, do they need their bill? But also, what about that guy in the corner who is acting like he wants to pinch my butt, is he serious? Is the woman with him going to be mad at me and make him leave a low tip (tips are about half the earnings of food servers)? Discretion is important—if the servers are busy, they can't be seen to watch the customers, since any glance can be interpreted as a sign of availability for service. They have to look only at the customer they are serving at the moment, while being aware that another is signalling to them for coffee.

They also have to manage their relations with the kitchen. Is it the right time to remind the kitchen about the steak order? Is the cook in a nasty enough mood to treat a reminder as a reason to forget the order completely?

And food servers have to keep an overview of the restaurant—given the number of customers and who is working in the kitchen, is now the right time to take orders for desserts so they will arrive in time, or is it too early for customers to think about dessert?[5]

Eve observed the work for several shifts, using some ergonomics software to note their movements. She noticed that the women and men had different walking patterns, even though they had the same job title and task assignments. Women serving food took 83 percent more steps per minute than the men assigned to exactly the same jobs in the same restaurants (see Table 4.1). Yes, it's true, women's legs are shorter on average and we take smaller steps, but the steps are only 10 percent smaller, so the difference in the number of steps was way more than could be explained by the sex difference in step length.[6] What was stranger was that even though the women were walking much faster than the men, they also walked during more of the time, so they were covering almost three times

Table 4.1 Characteristics and working postures of 9 female and 3 male food servers in a restaurant in Quebec			
Average	Women (N=9)	Men (N=3)	Ratio M/F
Age (years)	33.5	33.9	1.01
Height (metres)[a]	1.61	1.74	1.08
Body mass index[b]	23.9	26.1	1.09
% of work time spent standing[c]	72.4	84.8	1.17
% of work time spent walking[d]	27.4	15.1	0.55
Steps/minute during walking[e]	38.4	21.0	0.55
Steps at a time without stopping[f]	5.5	3.5	0.64

a Difference statistically significant at 0.001 level, t test.
b Body mass index (BMI) is calculated as (weight in kilograms) / (height in metres^2). Healthy BMI is thought to be between 18.5 and 25. Difference statistically significant at 0.05 level, t test.
c Difference statistically significant at 0.10 level, t test.
d Difference statistically significant at 0.10 level, t test.
e Difference statistically significant at 0.05 level, t test.
f Difference statistically significant at 0.01 level, t test.

Source: Calculated from Eve Laperrière, Suzy Ngomo, Marie-Christine Thibault, and Karen Messing, "Indicators for Choosing an Optimal Mix of Major Working Postures," *Applied Ergonomics* 37,3 (2006), 349–57.

the men's distance during their shifts. And all this extra walking had its costs. When Eve analyzed her questionnaire results, she found that women reported significantly more foot and ankle pain than men.[7]

Eve also wondered about male-female differences in strength. She remembered that when she was working in restaurants, the dishes were too big and too heavy; it seemed that the managers who chose the dishes were thinking about aesthetics rather than the health of their wait staff. Also, in many restaurants, including the ones she was observing, management shunned trays because they took too much space that could be used for revenue-producing tables. Servers had to pile up dishes against their bodies during transport.

So Eve's questionnaire asked about techniques for carrying dishes, and women said they carried multiple dishes in one hand significantly less often than men did. Smaller hands and weaker upper-body muscles could partly explain why the women had to scurry around more: they could carry less at a time, so they might be making more trips back and forth to the kitchen.

Thus, biological sex differences could partly explain why women had to do more walking. But we could also imagine some reasons related to gender roles: women could be running around more because they were more attentive to customers' requests, or because customers felt freer to ask them to get more items, or because they were given extra tasks by management. Significantly more women than men reported giving a greater priority to swift service than to protecting their arms and shoulders. Since customers appear to tip women less generously, women may need to service more customers in order to earn as much as men.[8] In addition, the responses to Eve's questionnaire showed that women reported doing more "housekeeping" tasks like refilling salt and pepper shakers (Table 4.2).

In summary—women and men with the same jobs in the same restaurants were being assigned different tasks, were to some extent performing different manipulations, and were therefore not using their bodies the same way at work. And women were suffering from more health symptoms.[9]

Segregation of tasks also occurs in industry. Tasks on assembly

Table 4.2 Some differences in task assignments between women and men		
Workplace example	Women's work involves	Men's work involves
Assembly line[a]	Extremely fast repetitive movements, more than 20 per minute, like packing objects in boxes	Repetitive movements not usually above 2 per minute, like loading boxes into a truck
Cleaning[b]	Handling weights up to 2 kg, like wastebaskets	Handling heavier weights, like vacuum cleaners
Food processing[c]	Trimming tiny pieces of extra fat off turkey breasts with a small knife	Killing turkeys and cutting them into big pieces with a big knife
Grocery stores[d]	Cashier—keying in food prices, prolonged static standing	Store clerk—Placing heavy items on display, walking from one department to another

a Barbara A. Silverstein, Larry J. Fine, and Thomas J. Armstrong, "Hand Wrist Cumulative Trauma Disorders in Industry," *British Journal of Industrial Medicine* 43 (1986), 779–84.

b K. Messing, C. Chatigny, J. Courville, "'Light' and 'Heavy' Work in the Housekeeping Service of a Hospital," *Applied Ergonomics* 29,6 (1998), 451–9.

c Nicole Vézina, Julie Courville, and Lucie Geoffrion, "Problèmes musculo-squelettiques, caractéristiques des postes de travailleurs et des postes de travailleuses sur une chaîne de découpe de dinde," in *Invisible: Issues in Women's Occupational Health and Safety / Invisible: La santé des travailleuses*, ed. Karen Messing, Barbara Neis, and Lucie Dumais (Charlottetown, PE: Gynergy Books, 1995), 29–61.

d Nicole Vézina, Céline Chatigny, and Karen Messing, "Un poste de manutention : symptômes et conditions de travail chez les caissières de deux supermarchés," *Maladies chroniques au Canada* 15,1 (1994), 19–24.

lines tend to be divided along gender lines, with women and men in jobs with different kinds of physical demands. In a cookie factory, Lucie Dumais and her colleagues found male assembly line workers running the big mixing machine and the ovens, while women were assigned to manually wrapping the cookies and putting the packages in small boxes. Men then packed the small boxes into bigger boxes, men loaded them into trucks, and men drove off with them.[10]

These task differences can lead to exposures relevant for occupational health. France Labrèche and her colleagues have found that women and men are not always exposed to the same cancer-causing chemicals, even within the same job title.[11] And an Australian group has shown that women do more repetitive work than men with the same job titles in the same companies.[12] Thus the men's and women's risk of cancer or musculoskeletal disorders can differ, even within the same job.

In my first three chapters, I have described some of our attempts to help women's committees end job segregation by gender. We were not very successful—in all three cases it could be argued that despite their economic advancement, ending or limiting job segregation turned out to be bad for women's health. The women technicians and older cleaners left their jobs, and the women health care aides were exhausted and injured from lifting patients. Is that generally true? Is maintaining job segregation by gender good for women's health? Before trying to answer that question, I need to describe how segregation works in jobs with a physical component.

In our research, gender segregation of tasks in low-wage work with a physical component often looks like what we see in Table 4.2.

The physical demands in women's jobs tend to look unimpressive, and women themselves have trouble making the case that their work is difficult. Thus, the fact of the tasks being different is not the problem; it is the lack of respect for what women do. But CINBIOSE researchers Nicole Vézina and Julie Courville compared weights manipulated by men in manual materials handling and by women sewing machine operators. The men lifted about 51 rolls of plastic a day. The rolls were heavy, about 18 kilograms each, and they were lifted using bars that weighed over 7 kilograms each. Since the rolls had to be manipulated more than once, the men ended up lifting 2,612 kilograms per day, an impressive amount and not at all easy on their backs. The women, on the other hand, had to sew relatively light pieces of cloth together. Each piece of cloth weighed about 265 grams, only about 1 percent of the weight of each plastic roll. So, each time the women lifted the pants, they exerted relatively little effort. But since they put together 1,869 pairs of pants in a day, they ended up lifting about a third more weight than the men, for a total of 3,486 kilograms. And their feet were also pushing heavy, badly maintained pedals on the sewing machines for a total of over 16,000 kilograms of forceful exertion.[13] The physical consequences of these different kinds of demands are not directly comparable, but we do know that the sewing machine operators were suffering from shoulder problems.

Although both women's and men's tasks in maintenance and industry are repetitive, women's are generally much more repetitive, with a faster pace. Men handle heavier weights and use more machines.[14] But the gender stereotyping depends on context. When the heavy weights to be handled are people, in health care or preschool, women lift them.[15] When the machines are sewing machines, women use them. Women are more commonly exposed to prolonged standing in one place, whereas men move around more.[16] Women cleaners stretch, crouch, and bend more than male cleaners.[17] Canadian men work 5.8 hours per week more than women at a paid job and way outnumber women among those working more than 40 hours per week,[18] while women do more unpaid domestic work.[19]

This segregation is pervasive and persistent. In 1941, women were 22 percent of the Canadian workforce,[20] climbing to 47 percent in 2020.[21] But women's and men's professions are still different: only two of the ten most common women's job titles (retail sales clerks and restaurant help) are among the ten most common for men (Table 4.3).[22] In Canada, for women and men to be distributed evenly throughout the labour force, about half would have to change jobs.[23] During the COVID-19 pandemic, women (especially racial-

Table 4.3 Top 10 professions for women and men, Canada, 2016		
	Women	Men
1	Retail salespersons	Transport truck drivers
2	Registered nurses and registered psychiatric nurses	Retail salespersons
3	Cashiers	Retail and wholesale trade managers
4	Elementary school and kindergarten teachers	Janitors, caretakers, and building superintendents
5	Administrative assistants	Construction trades helpers and labourers
6	Food counter attendants, kitchen helpers, and related support occupations	Automotive service technicians, truck and bus mechanics, and mechanical repairers
7	Administrative officers	Material handlers
8	Nurse aides, orderlies, and patient service associates	Carpenters
9	General office support workers	Food counter attendants, kitchen helpers, and related support occupations
10	Early childhood educators and assistants	Cooks

Source: Statistics Canada, Census of Population, 2016.

ized women) turned out to hold about 76 percent of the most exposed jobs, such as the "essential" health care and cashier jobs.[24] Women were consequently reported to be 73 percent of infected health care workers.[25]

At lower educational/income levels, where the physical components of jobs are more obvious, jobs are even more segregated. In 2011, 60 percent of Canadian women and 73 percent of men between twenty-five and thirty-four had no university degree. For these young men and women to be distributed evenly across the workforce, statisticians calculate that 62 percent of workers would have to change jobs.[26]

All this boils down to the fact that women at the low end of the job market work at tasks where the physical demands are different from those in men's jobs. We have seen that when women try to enter men's jobs or do the same tasks as men, they encounter physical and social obstacles. So why don't women just try to get recognition for the tasks they do and the physical proficiency they have?

Easier said than done.

Are women more prone to get sick than men?

Florence Chappert is an energetic, practical engineer who was put in charge of gender-related activities at the French National Agency for Improving Working Conditions (ANACT).[27] She supervised an ergonomic intervention at a large print shop whose managers had decided not to hire women anymore since, they argued, too many women were complaining of musculoskeletal disorders induced by their work. Almost all the women workers were assigned to the section where books were assembled, so Florence asked the ANACT ergonomists to observe the work of the 26 women and 37 men in that section.[28]

The ergonomists made four major observations. First, the women's task assignments within the section were very different from the men's; seven of the ten tasks were done only by one gender (Table 4.4). The women were asked to handle the books one by one, whereas the men serviced machines. Second, the task demands in the women's work were very heavy and becoming heavier. The

Table 4.4 Job assignments by gender in book printing and assembly in France, 2012			
Job	Women	Men	% Women
Assistant binder	17	7	71
Machine operator	1	14	7
Assistant operator	–	4	–
Finisher	3	1	75
Foreman	–	3	–
Conductor	–	3	–
Materials handler	–	3	–
Trimmer	–	2	–
Clerk	2	–	100
Sewing machine operator	3	–	100
Total	26	37	41

Source: Florence Chappert, Karen Messing, Eric Peltier, and Jessica Riel, "Conditions de travail et parcours dans l'entreprise : vers une transformation qui intègre l'ergonomie et le genre?," *Revue multidisciplinaire sur l'emploi, le syndicalisme et le travail* (REMEST) 9,2 (2014), 46–67, www.erudit.org.

women had handled about 1,500 books per hour in 1972, but 8,000 books per hour in 2009, while the number of women workers had not risen anywhere near to the same extent. Third, the task demands in the men's jobs had become lighter over the same period, since their jobs were increasingly mechanized. Finally, the men tended to leave the book assembling section very rapidly, either promoted out or leaving for greener pastures. The ergonomists concluded that probably the women were suffering more injuries than the men, just because they were staying longer at more taxing work.

When the ergonomists gave their report on gendered task demands to the workers and managers, the women wept, because their state of exhaustion and pain had finally been acknowledged. They had never dared to ask to be promoted to the easier jobs held by the men, but at least now the ergonomists had shown how hard their jobs were. Unfortunately, afraid of the men's reaction, the managers refused to take action to change the task assignments.

Only after the ANACT ergonomists persisted were they finally able to make some small changes in the women's task assignments and workload, although workplace segregation was never really challenged. When it was all over, Florence Chappert described the intensity of the taboos surrounding gender inequalities in these terms (my translation):

> Companies find it hard to treat these questions of gender and equality directly. They don't want to leave themselves open to affirmative action and they are convinced that they have already achieved equality . . . When we discuss these issues with the [joint union-management committees concerned with occupational health and safety], we have to show them our numbers to convince them that the health inequalities really exist—and the realization is often brutal! That's why we have developed strategies [to return

our results to industry] that allow them to assimilate these data progressively, because if we don't, they are too hard to accept.

Florence's description of the resistance of employers and colleagues reminds me of so many of our studies in Quebec. Revealing the hidden physical requirements imposed on women in food service, banking, office work, teaching, and hotel housekeeping has, by and large, not been sufficient to improve their lot, although some of these groups have been galvanized by the research results and have led successful strikes that have improved their working conditions and/or their pay. The women crying, the fact that there is a taboo protecting job and task segregation, all this intense resistance arouses my feminist instincts. What are the powerful forces behind the taboo? Where exactly does the task segregation come from? Is it justified by biological differences between women and men, or are there other reasons for it? Is there a better way to protect the health of women and men than by assigning them to different tasks?

The next chapter examines the biological basis for job segregation.

5.
SAME, DIFFERENT, OR UNDERSTUDIED?

n 2015, an international meeting of feminist researchers—le Congrès international des recherches féministes dans la francophonie—came to Montreal and asked me to give one of their keynote lectures. I found myself in a big hall surrounded by hundreds of social science researchers, many of whom knew a lot more than me about women and their jobs. There were three themes: think, create, and act—I hoped I was meant to be "action" and that no one expected a biologist to be at home with social theory.

I told the audience some stories about bodies and the workplace, like the ones I have told here. I wanted feminist researchers to consider the implications of their studies for both gender equality and women's health. I asked them to think about whether, sometimes, job segregation could possibly protect women's health, even while posing serious problems for gender equality. I told about some of the difficulties women like the communications technicians face when they enter jobs previously occupied only by men: that, in addition to stereotyping and harassment, women were at extra risk of work accidents and musculoskeletal disorders due to tasks designed for the body of the average male worker. I described working with local unions to find solutions.

During the question period, a young researcher from the Democratic Republic of Congo identified herself. She questioned my whole message: "In *The Second Sex*, Simone de Beauvoir told us, 'One is not born a woman, but becomes one.' She meant that biology does not define women. Are you telling me that she was wrong?" I think she was saying that biological differences of chromosomal origin—"sex differences"—might be of little importance in determining what happens to women in the workplace. In the two minutes available at the end of a long session, I stumbled over my tongue and gave an incoherent, incomplete response. I was disappointed with myself, so I went home and thought about what I could have said; those reflections gave rise to this book.

Many, many feminist health scientists and union activists share the concerns of that young woman. They are worried about gender discrimination and see an emphasis on biological sex differences as encouraging stereotyping and thus inequality. As a researcher in biology, I see three issues:

> Are there biological differences that are relevant to job assignments and job design?
> If so, are the differences big and important enough that they can affect women's occupational health? If they are not taken into account, does that mean all jobs will be designed only for men's biology, and women will get sick or injured?
> Are there scientific solutions that can preserve equality and women's health?

Biological differences between women and men

The extent of male-female biological differences is a complicated and critical question, not only for feminists, but also for natural scientists.[1] I have heard the position that I will call "sameness" that says that people come in various versions that are plastic and not strongly associated with a single sex/gender. Those I will call "difference" feminists believe there are important ways that women differ from men throughout their lives. In the workplace, these two points of view come with different risks and advantages for women and men, for manual and non-manual workers. What I am calling "sameness" arguments could imply that gender, or social role, is relevant to disease prevention and biological sex is less so—that whether people have one or two X chromosomes has little bearing on the health effects of their jobs, task assignments, or work activities. I am calling "difference" arguments those that might imply that women's and men's job and task assignments should be conditioned by data on biological vulnerability; men or women should be assigned to jobs and tasks suited to their sex-specific strengths.[2]

These opposing positions, which appear theoretical, have led to practical difficulties in favouring women's health at work. Should we publicize, emphasize, or conceal women's higher accident rate in male-dominated jobs? Should we call on toxicologists, industrial hygienists, and ergonomists to study what may be sex-specific physiology underlying occupational risks that affect women much more often than men—such as musculoskeletal disorders, "sick building syndrome," chronic fatigue syndrome, and fibromyalgia—or should we just study the diseases as diseases? Should we explore whether women and men should be assigned different limits for lifting weights? for chemical exposures? Is it a good idea to employ women to warn other workers in jobs where toxic chemicals can be smelled, given our higher olfactory sensitivity?[3] Should we favour legislation to adapt jobs specifically for pregnant women or should we imitate some US policymakers in treating pregnancy like "any other temporary disability"? And what should we do about people transitioning between sexes/genders, since there has been little to no research on the influence of exogenous sex hormones on reactions to workplace toxins?[4]

My own approach, as a biologist, is to concentrate on the biological mechanisms involved in each of these issues, while not forgetting the social context.

Sex differences and job design

Let's start with the science. What follows is a greatly simplified presentation of the contribution of genes to sex differences.[5] The emphasis is on identifying the biological differences that are important and not easy to change, and that need to be accommodated in the workplace. Anyone who wants to know more should read Anne Fausto-Sterling's articles and books on the difficulties of identifying sex differences in socially relevant characteristics[6] and Springer, Stellman, and Jordan-Young on how to think about sex differences.[7]

Genes, chromosomes, and the workplace

During my original training in genetics years ago, I learned how people with two X chromosomes, by definition women,[8] develop female reproductive systems from embryonic bumps and folds at an early stage of development, starting at about the sixth week of fetal life. I was fascinated by the fact that men, with one large X chromosome and one small Y chromosome, develop male reproductive systems from the same bumps and folds.[9] In other words, the presence or

Figure 5.1 Development of biological sex from genetic sex

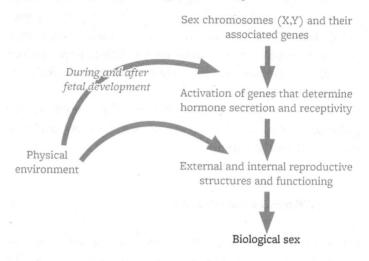

absence of a very few genes on the Y chromosome, the number of copies and the state of a few genes on the X chromosome, are usually responsible for what is technically called sexual dimorphism, or male-female average differences in size, body proportions, and functioning (Figure 5.1).[10] Already during fetal life, and later during childhood, the environment interacts with these genes to produce adaptations in some physical structures and in metabolism.[11] Women and men end up not only with bodies that usually look different, but with bodies that produce hormones, perceive some stimuli, and metabolize food and pollutants in somewhat different ways.

Since these differences contribute to some of the obstacles women face in the workplace, I will briefly summarize them. It is important to note here that genetic sex is not the same as biological sex. That is, genes don't work alone to create women's and men's bodies. Biological sex includes body shape and size, proportion of muscles, reproductive experience, hormone administration, and

Figure 5.2 Development of gender from biological sex assigned at birth

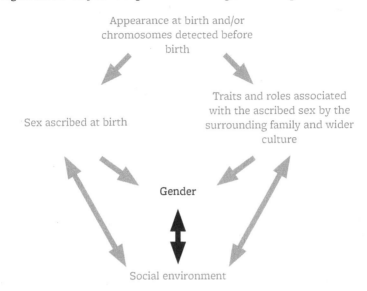

metabolism. A woman can have two standard X chromosomes but have a body that doesn't look or act "typically" female, depending not only on her other genes, but also on what she eats, drinks, and works with, or what else she does with her body, like sleeping or exercising, or what she wants to look like. And those behaviours are conditioned by her social influences and by her self-identification as a girl or woman, known as gender (Figure 5.2).

Gender and biological sex influence each other. All her life, a person who identifies as female (whatever her chromosomes may be) will have a series of experiences that influence her gender and her biology, and help determine what becomes of her mind and body (Figure 5.3). So, a young woman who (exceptionally in North America) is encouraged to develop her muscles will end up with a body that looks more "male" by North American standards. This perception may then cause people to ascribe male gender stereo-

Figure 5.3 Biological sex evolves over the lifetime

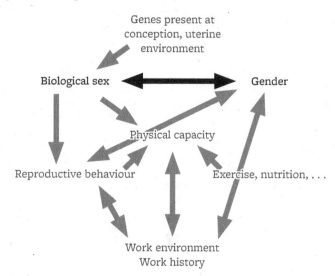

types to her. One has just to look at various trolls' comments on tennis champion Serena Williams's body to understand how biological differences and similarities deriving from physical training can influence gender stereotyping.[12]

A word of warning. Almost all of the biological differences I will describe here are changeable and many are small.

Size and shape

Men are, on average, taller and heavier than women. In the Canadian army population, about 8 percent taller and 26 percent heavier.[13] But women are not just small men; we are shaped differently (Table 5.1). When I went to the Ontario Science Centre a few years ago, someone had set up an exhibit with four points painted on a mattress pad. You were supposed to put your hands on the front ones and your knees on the back ones. One by one, I watched women and men go into position and, I admit it, giggled, as all of the men, but none of the women, fell forward on their noses. Women's centre of mass in that position is significantly further back than men's. But we have to stop laughing at men's centre of mass when we get on bicycles or drive landscaping tractors. Not only are the dimensions of these machines generally too big for many women, but badly designed equipment can position us in a way that puts more pressure on our shoulders and backs. And, in the case of bicycles, on our genital area.

Fat accounts for about 25 percent of white North American women's average body weight but 15 percent of white men's. Women have more subcutaneous fat and less fat in the abdominal cavity ("visceral fat"). Women have breasts and, from the waist down, are

Table 5.1 Body size of female and male Canadian Armed Forces personnel, 2012			
	Female	Male	Ratio M/F
Buttock–knee length (mm)	582	615	1.06
Chest circumference (mm)	941	1,054	1.12
Sitting height (mm)	873	930	1.07
Stature (mm)	1,638	1,769	1.08
Waist circumference (mm)	863	951	1.10
Weight (kg)	69	87	1.26

Source: Allan Keefe and Harry Angel, 2012 *Canadian Forces Anthropometric Survey (CFAS) Final Report* (Ottawa: Defence Research and Development Canada, 2015), 47–50.
Note: These were the best data I could find, but please note that 92% of women and 93% of men measured in this study were "Caucasian," much higher than the proportion in the general population. Also, army personnel are younger and in better health than the general population.

generally more pear-shaped, while men are shaped more like apples.[14] (The dimensions of African American women and men are said to resemble each other more closely, but racialized groups have been seriously understudied and I have been unable to find reliable data—and nothing at all on First Nations.) Men have bigger waists, but their hip measurements are similar to women's, so their waists indent less. These differences have implications for design—for example, tool belts designed for men, when they are not too big for us, can dig uncomfortably into women's hips, and this is what we hear from working women. Women's proportionally wider hips can often translate into an accentuated angle between the thighbone and the lower leg (quadriceps angle or "Q angle"), possibly contributing to more knee problems among women athletes[15] and, again, possibly important for other professions, like boot design for technicians who climb utility poles.

I need to emphasize again that few of these differences are absolute. There is almost always overlap between the dimensions of the largest women and those of smaller men, and almost all of the research has been done on white people of European origin or has not made ethnic differences visible. (The lack of information on size and shape of women and non-white populations turned out to be a big problem when adjusted face masks were needed during the COVID-19 pandemic.) And I have seen no physiological or anthropometric studies on the various non-binary or trans populations.

Sex differences in bone shapes may be trivial, and they are usually far outweighed by similarities. The fact that the top of the lower leg bone (tibia) is shaped differently in women and men[16] and that women's feet may be narrower in proportion to their length[17] may contribute little to the sex/gender difference in marathon times and in lower limb disorders. Although we can't even be sure of this, because scientists haven't studied it enough. So we don't know what design changes are necessary so that shoes, clothing, and floor surfaces can be adapted for all women and men. We can be sure, though, that running tracks, tennis courts, and industrial workplaces, tools, and equipment are only slowly being designed with women's (or non-white) bodies and proportions in mind, because these populations weren't allowed to use them in the early days and because the subject hasn't interested many researchers (see chapter 12 for some of the technical/scientific obstacles).

Strength

Most people would agree with the statement that men are stronger than women. But feminists (and employers and unions and policy-makers) would like to know more. What strength? Are all muscles the same? All movements? In all positions? At all speeds? What happens if women are trained as much as men? What would have happened if I had ignored my father and continued with the broad jump—could I have continued to outjump the boys? What about the persistence of strength over time? Do women and men fatigue at the same rate? Do we experience muscle pain the same way?

Unfortunately, once again, most of the research on load manipulation has been done with white male subjects only and on the types of loads that people manipulate in jobs usually done by men. Relatively little research has been done on the wiggly loads women tend to lift at work (children, hospital patients) and the strengths women more often need (ability to stand still for long periods, to shift smaller weights in more awkward positions, like grocery purchases for cashiers or small obstreperous children for daycare workers). We have not studied such questions as how women can best carry loads in front of us or how we balance loads on our backs. At all. The little research that includes women most often comes from the military in countries like the US, Canada, and Israel, who are studying highly selected, young populations that may not be typical of manual workers. I have to add that sometimes our military research appears to paint sex differences with an unduly broad brush, generalizing from little data.[18]

Still, we can be reasonably sure that men show more strength while doing most tasks but that the type of strength varies between women and men. André Plamondon's research group has found that even inexperienced men can force themselves to lift boxes twice as heavy as those women can force themselves to lift (139 kilograms versus 68 kilograms),[19] even women who do this kind of work for a living. Women's muscles react to lifting a 6-kilogram load in much the same way as men's when they lift a 12-kilogram load,[20] although we deploy our shoulder muscles in somewhat different ways.[21] There is a bigger sex difference in average upper-body strength (50 percent) than in the legs (30 percent),[22] so sex differences are more obvious in weight lifting than in walking or kicking.

And when it comes to endurance, the advantage tends to go in the opposite direction. There are two broad types of muscle fibres: Type I or slow-twitch fibres are associated with sustained contractions or endurance under aerobic (oxygen available) conditions, and women and long-distance joggers have proportionally more. Type II or fast-twitch fibres are associated with intense contractions under anaerobic (oxygen-depleted) conditions, and men and sprinters have proportionally more of them.[23] Strength training of the weightlifting type tends to increase both types of fibres among both women and men.[24] The differences in fibre types may explain in part why women's and men's performance on many strength-related tasks tend to converge as the task duration gets longer.[25] In other words, women are relatively better at endurance than at short bursts of speed. There is a much bigger sex difference for lifting weights ("explosive" force, using more type II fibres) than for carrying weights (endurance, using more type I fibres).

I should mention again that we have no idea whether the strength differences come from hormones, from some other sex-differentiated gene function,[26] or from training effects. I have not seen any longitudinal studies of the strength of young people as they transition from one sex to the other, although a trans friend told me he gradually became able to lift heavier and heavier weights as his testosterone levels increased.

Julie Côté, an expert in biomechanics, does research on gender, sex, and work. She has been exploring why women report more pain than men. Some of her results point to different patterns of muscle activation among women and men using their shoulder muscles to do the same task, with women's tending toward more repetitive use of the same fibres, possibly because they work closer to their physiological limits.[27] In an intriguing paper, Côté also tells us that women's proprioception (sense of their body in space) is different, with women tending to experience their bodies as smaller than they really are while men experience theirs as closer to their true size.[28] However, she emphasizes that there is always variability among women and among men as well as overlap in the performance of the two sexes.[29]

So there are not only sex/gender differences in lifting strength, there seem to be sex/gender differences or at least variations by sex/gender in how the body handles a number of types of movements. There are also sex differences in how pain is processed, at least in mice. (See the more extensive discussion of gender/sex differences in pain in chapter 11.) These are matters for serious interest, given the numerous research results showing a much higher accident and injury rate for women in male-dominated manual jobs and in the military, and a higher rate of musculoskeletal disorders among women workers in all kinds of jobs.

Among the many things we don't know: We have no idea how far training could go to improve women's lifting strength, given that training can improve muscle but not necessarily the other structures involved in lifting, like the ligaments and tendons that connect muscles with bones and joints. Aside from a few studies by Plamondon's team,[30] we don't know much about how to adapt weightlifting techniques to women's body shapes and muscle fibre types. We haven't inventoried the ways that women with experience in non-traditional jobs adapt their tools, equipment, and techniques. We don't know whether such adaptation would improve the health of women manual workers or just make them work closer to their physiological limit.[31] And biomechanics experts point out that the optimal ways to use female and male bodies may be different and if so, work site design needs to be rethought.[32]

Pregnancy and menstrual cycles

Managers like reliable employees who show up every day in the same state and do their job in the way they always have. Pregnant women are a pain in the neck. They go to the bathroom a lot, they get increasingly tired, and as their bodies get more cumbersome, they can't always do the same tasks in the same way. On top of that, their exposures to toxins in the workplace can seriously affect fetuses, making employers worry about being held responsible. But employers in most countries aren't allowed to just fire these burdensome workers. In Quebec and many other jurisdictions, pregnant workers are eligible for "accommodation," or job reassignments, because their fetuses can't be exposed to dangerous levels of chemicals or noise.

In theory, the law also protects pregnant women from exposure to conditions that would injure them because of their pregnant state, although in practice the law is almost always invoked to protect the fetus. As one charming physician testifying for an employer put it, "The problem is that the pregnant worker has a member of the public in her womb" (who he presumably thinks is entitled to more protection than the mom).[33] But we do need to think about pregnant women's circulatory, respiratory, and musculoskeletal systems that are doing extra work and shouldn't be overtaxed. In later stages of pregnancy, women's new size and shape may need different spaces or redesigned tools. And all this has to happen without being unfair to colleagues who are not pregnant. I say this because in Quebec, despite our wonderful law providing most pregnant women with an adjusted workload, employers can still put the burden of these adjustments on their non-pregnant colleagues.[34]

Reproductive involvement of women continues after childbirth, and Quebec women do about seven hours more domestic work per week than men, nine hours more if children are young.[35] (This is, of course, not a biological difference between women and men, but does possibly derive in part from the fact that women can nurse infants and most men can't.) This extended workday can interact with the physical and cognitive work to produce fatigue and health problems.[36]

Some working conditions affect women's reproduction specifically—the menstrual cycle itself can be lengthened, shortened, or made irregular or more painful by exposure to solvents, cold, or some work schedules.[37] Some employers don't see why they would have to adjust to these personal, private problems. However, employers have always had to respond to employees' other "personal" needs. North American laws, regulations, and policy require employers to provide toilets, drinking water, lunch breaks, rest periods, and reasonable time off for sleeping and family time. Is it only the "second bodies" whose personal needs are seen as illegitimate?

Scientists are like employers in that they want their research subjects to show up in the same state every day. But women have cycles and pregnancies and then we have menopause. So historically, before women insisted on being included in biomedical research and forced the creation of the Canadian Institute of Gender and Health,[38] scientists refused or forgot to include female animals or humans in their investigations.[39] And yes, some science says women's ability to tolerate pain, heat,[40] and muscular effort[41] can vary over the menstrual cycle, and scientists have made a case for there being variability in reactions in both males and females.[42] Data are still missing on all these questions about biomechanics, and the situation is even worse in toxicology.

Other possible biological differences related to workplace exposures

It was twenty years ago, in 2001, that the US Institute of Medicine assembled a committee to examine sex differences in biology. In their 288-page report, there were about ten pages on metabolism.[43] In 2017, a toxicologist published a review of what is known and not known about sex differences in metabolism of toxic substances in the human environment.[44] In 2012, Donna Mergler gave a lecture asking toxicologists for study of potential sex differences in effects of environmental chemicals on the brain, supplying several examples where females and males seem to metabolize chemicals somewhat differently. But so far, nobody much has stepped up to the plate; a large number of studies still exclude women, use only male animals, or do not identify the sex of their subjects.[45]

One of the reasons for thinking about female-male differences in toxin metabolism is that many toxins interact with hormones. An obvious example is "endocrine disruptors," a class of pesticides and other environmental contaminants that can be found in some workplaces and that interact with hormones. Also, many toxins affect and are affected by body fats, and women and men have different proportions of energy-storing "white" fat (men have more) to energy-burning "brown" fat (women have more).[46] This is important because most exposure standards have been established by experiments with only male animals or only men.

Another physiological difference between the average American woman and man probably stems from women's smaller size. At the same external temperature reading, women feel colder[47] and perform less well on certain mental tasks.[48] It is not surprising that workers in large offices can disagree about where the thermostat should be set.

Adapting the workplace for women

Broadly, "difference" feminists should want more to be known about female-male differences in strength, physiology, toxin metabolism, pain experience, and reproductive biology, among other chromosomally influenced phenomena. They point to the fact that women were more likely to die from heart attacks before doctors learned that women's heart attacks were "atypical," that is, not like men's.[49] These feminists would then want to struggle so that the differences would be recognized in the workplace and so that the recognition would contribute to workplace design, labour standards, and regulations. They would emphasize the importance of diversity in making up work teams.

But "sameness" feminists maintain that politically and scientifically, "difference" feminists have got it wrong. As Simone de Beauvoir's statement implies, gender stereotyping exaggerates difference and tends to freeze women and men into rigid roles whose requirements vary enormously over time and space, unjustified by any dichotomy in chromosomal determination. So "sameness" feminists don't see why we should emphasize sex differences rather than similarities. And it is true, from a biologist's point of view, that men's and women's performance and functioning are not completely different. Few of even the well-established differences are universal. Some women are taller than almost all men, and some men are smaller than almost all women. Some women are relatively impervious to pain and some men are hypersensitive. And some people reject being defined as either women or men, so how would they be considered if sex/gender were to be used to define labour standards?

Lawyers have argued that Canadian law gives employers a duty to protect women (specifically) from harm while giving them equal access to employment.[50] Ergonomists would say that if equipment, job requirements, and job design were adapted and adjustable for all, male-female differences would be irrelevant. After all, some people need glasses to help them see or sticks to help them walk. The degree and amount of male/female differences in manipulating objects depend on all kinds of parameters of the work situation that can potentially be adjusted.[51] When one of the only women in a machine shop with over a thousand men was asked to tighten bolts on a diesel engine, it took her a while to realize she needed a longer wrench. When she used the same-length wrench, she took 40 percent *longer* to tighten the bolts than her male partner; when she got a wrench twice as long, she was *faster than him* by 60 percent.[52] The longer wrench gave her a mechanical advantage that meant she could exert less force, even though she had to move the handle through a longer distance. Her measured grip strength was less than half that of her male co-workers' and about one-third of her male partner's, yet, given the right tool, she could do the task more quickly than he.

Sex-associated differences in comfortable temperatures, tool grip sizes, or desirable desk heights cost money to accommodate—locally adjustable temperatures, a wider range of tools, desks or chairs that go up and down. And management approaches will have to be built from scratch to deal with menstrual cycle effects such as those resulting from work schedule variations or cold temperatures. Not an easy task, given the reluctance of employers to spend much money on workplace improvements.

So, given all these differences, and given scientists' and employers' lack of interest in women's occupational health, job segregation may now play a role in protecting women's health. But it is certainly dangerous for gender equality in the workplace.

How can we move this along?

Toward solutions

I think the "sameness" feminists are right in maintaining that women and men are not different species and that women and men have a huge, overlapping range of cognitive, physical, and emotional characteristics. I agree with other feminist scientists like Anne Fausto-Sterling and Jeanne Stellman that biological differences between women and men are generated not only by chromosomes but also by gendered experiences and gender inequality involving diet, exercise, aesthetic norms, time use, and many other parts of life. I respect the findings of Ruth Hubbard and Anne Fausto-Sterling who say that many people with either XX or XY chromosomal makeup can still not be biologically defined unequivocally as belonging exclusively to one sex.

I therefore agree that chromosomal sex or even gender identity should not determine job and task assignments in the workplace. But I think the "difference" people are right in admitting that sex-related physiology plays a part in what makes most people calling themselves "women" different from most "men" in some respects that are relevant to occupational health.

I have to repeat that I am not at ease with the theoretical issues and I'll leave them to feminists more at ease with theory. I'm sure they will agree with me that the communications technicians, cleaners, and health care aides need change now. What will help? To make the workplace safe and equitable for women and men, we can help to push for three changes: more information, a better approach to human resources, and, especially, tighter bonds among women workers (and their allies).

More information: I think that to make the political struggle work for low-paid women in jobs with physical components, we need to ask some practical questions. Is this or that task adapted for women's bodies? How can we make it better? What are women's bodies really like, and how do they experience their situation in the workplace right now? How could designers improve women's work? We also need to identify the mechanisms at play—our approach will be different if women show more reactions to solvent exposure because of hormonal interactions compared to the situation where, being shorter, women find their noses are positioned closer to open pots of paint. In a word, we need more scientific and technical knowledge (see chapters 10 to 12).

A note on what happens now. At best, ergonomists and engineers say that they want physical jobsite dimensions and requirements to be such that 95 percent of workers will be able to do those jobs. In my business we often hear about those happy 95 percent. But, in practice, that may mean that the job can be done by 95 percent but only a minority of those 95 percent are comfortable, more often men. So we need a wider variety of tools and equipment as well as greater access to adjustable furniture.

Workplace policy: We can see all of the differences described above as deficiencies of one sex or the other, or we can see them as sources of diverse advantages and talents. In a decent human resources environment, the employer will be looking to create and nurture a team with complementary skills and an environment where people can work in partnership.[53] Male firefighters have told me they don't want women on their teams because they want someone big to drag them out of the fire if they inhale too many fumes. But they are the first to say that they don't spend all their time dragging their colleagues' bodies around. Firefighting teams need to have some big, strong people, some little, fast people, and some fantastic strategic thinkers. Unfortunately, what we have seen when women enter male-dominated workplaces is that the women are encouraged to be more like the men who are already there. Unions need to work toward getting employers to take more responsibility for diversity so that they can reap the advantages of the added talents.

Solidarity: I think the millions of low-paid women who have suffered workplace oppression, accidents, and injuries might be tempted to say that neither denying nor highlighting sex differences has helped them. Whatever the biological differences turn out to be, *we no longer want to feel ashamed of our bodies in the workplace.* We don't want to hear jokes about our cycles, our periods, our menopause, or our boobs. We don't want to be thought of as having "different" or "atypical" bodies because many varieties of bodies are perfectly normal, including ours. We want the workplace to deal straightforwardly with women's bodies and our needs, just as they deal with men's bodies (not perfectly either, by the way).

Working women need to get together to insist on changes. Once women stop feeling ashamed of being women, we can start to defend our interests. If we can do it through a union, we get more protection and safety in numbers. More than theory, low-paid women workers need to demand practical interventions that take sex differences into account without exaggerating them and that result in both gender equality and health. They need to insist on workplaces adapted to their "second bodies" and committed to developing productive teamwork. Sometimes, that means adapting workplaces for a wider range of bodies, including women and men of various ages and ethnicities. Sometimes it means thinking really hard about team development. And sometimes, it means thinking about human differences, and how to accommodate and profit from them. We may have to go beyond individual workplaces and move to policy.

Policy changes

Women have always had to balance equality with health concerns. Historically, for example, women have faced uncomfortable choices in relation to night work.[54] Because women were thought weaker and because gender roles give women a major role in child care, many countries outlawed night work for women in factories. Some unions have asked for legislation to excuse women from night work. Science tells us that night work is not good for most people's health, since it interferes with the body's natural rhythms and may result in a propensity for obesity[55] and various diseases.[56] Mothers who work at night may find it especially hard to catch up on sleep during the day and they may accumulate harmful sleep deficits. So feminists should be happy when women's health is protected by night work laws.

Not so fast, though—sometimes, this type of law has kept women out of good jobs or high-paying shifts. And the laws are applied selectively—women in health care and some other stereotypically female night work jobs have not been "protected." Gender-specific laws can reinforce gender-stereotyped roles, making women more available to their families than men while decreasing women's access to economic equality, so maybe feminists should be against them.

Or, take exposure standards. Governments often ask ergonomists how much weight can be lifted by women versus men. And it is true that, at the same weight lifted, there are more physiological costs to almost all women than to most men. So many feminists would like different exposure limits and different pre-employment strength tests for women and men.[57] But would feminists really want the workplace to be effectively divided into two worlds, separate by sex? Wouldn't women be excluded from more jobs? And what would happen to smaller, weaker men or taller, stronger women? Would they want to change categories? Would there be a special category for non-binary workers?

Sex-based exposure standards would pose problems similar to those that come up from time to time in athletic competitions, where women who are "too" good at track and field have to submit to tests of "femaleness." The controversies about what is the "right" level of testosterone to permit among men or women athletes are complex and constantly evolve as we come to understand how bodies produce hormones and when and why they may over- or underproduce.[58] If we promulgated separate standards in other workplaces, would some women sue to be admitted to male standards to get higher pay? Would men ask to be admitted to female standards to protect their backs?

Anyway, right now we are very far from having the knowledge base to decide on any kind of exposure standard that could vary by sex/gender. And sex/gender is not the only determinant of physiological differences relevant to the workplace. Economic and social opportunities play a huge role in how human bodies develop,[59] and genes other than those relating to sex also determine physical attributes. Would we want to have different employment standards for immigrants of East Asian origin, who are generally shorter and slimmer than Europeans? Would we want to do DNA analysis of employees to decide on their acceptable exposures to chemicals as a function of the proportion of genes they might have from each continent?[60] But maybe we should just make and enforce more general labour standards, saying that employers need to adapt workplaces to everyone, and everyone should have equal access to employment. What would employers have to say about that?

How can we get employers to provide appropriate work environments? Our answer needs to be based not only on science, but also on organizational justice and political action. I have mentioned that a first step is that women have to stop being ashamed of our bodies. A second step is to point out the advantages of diversity and teamwork, and insist on adaptations in tools, equipment, and team building. The third step is to get together in solidarity and support each other. And the one right after that is to figure out how to transform the workplace, a scientific question as much as a political one. The next chapters will ask: How can or should we intervene so as to allow women equal access to jobs and remuneration without risking our health? What are the best strategies? Ergonomists at our research centre have taken two somewhat different approaches and we are wondering about how to go on from here.

PART III.
CHANGING THE
WORKPLACE

6.
RE-ENGINEERING WOMEN'S WORK

started off on the wrong foot in the 1970s when I began thinking about women's jobs. My UQAM colleague Donna Mergler had heard that Jeanne Stellman, then a chemist with the American Oil, Chemical and Atomic Workers union, would be giving a talk in Toronto on women and occupational health.[1] With an ergonomics consultant and two employees of the CSN labour union, we hopped excitedly on the train and found ourselves occupying seats face to face for the five-hour trip. We got into an argument that lasted almost the whole time.

The discussion was about how the unions should deal with male-female biological differences so as to promote equality at the same time as women's health. The most obvious example of a male-female biological difference is pregnancy, and working women in Quebec had recently acquired paid maternity leave. Now, the government was proposing to give pregnant or nursing women exposed to a risk for themselves, the fetus, or their nursing infant the right to leave their dangerous job at virtually full pay until the pregnancy, the nursing, or the danger was past.[2] All five of us women felt strongly about the new legislation. Two of us (the consultant and I) maintained that special leave for pregnant women exposed to dangers at work was unnecessary because almost any chemical or situation that was dangerous for pregnant women would be dangerous for men and non-pregnant women. We had some examples to back our idea, and we feared that special treatment would endanger women's access to jobs. The two union counsellors and Donna, who had been training workers in health and safety for years, maintained that some everyday conditions were so risky that pregnancy was sufficient to push the danger into an unacceptable zone. They thought that pregnant women were especially tired and overloaded and that their fetuses were at critical stages of development. They wanted women to get special consideration during pregnancy, so their health and their children's health would not suffer permanent damage.

I should have noticed that the three women who knew the most about pregnant workers were the ones who disagreed with me, but I stayed opposed to the protective legislation after the train took me home. I heard a rumour many years later, that my opposition had made it more difficult for the Quebec legislation to pass. After all, I was (then) an expert in genetics. But, as soon as the law passed, I did accept requests from the unions to train them in how to recognize risks for pregnant women, how to diminish the risks, and at what stage of pregnancy women should be withdrawn from a dangerous situation. So I had to listen to the women describe their working conditions. Conditions that surprised me, tough conditions. And slowly, listening to the pregnant women who lifted patients, sewed bras, and worked cash registers, I changed my mind. No, pregnant women especially shouldn't stand all day; no, they especially shouldn't run the risk of having fetuses deafened by noise or malformed by chemicals. No, they especially shouldn't be working night shifts. When work is difficult, pregnancy can push it over the line into horrible.

I also realized over time that I had been dead wrong about the effects on equality too. In the long run, politically, the legislation has turned out to be a gift to women in all sorts of ways. Protective pregnancy leave is still the only place where women are specifically considered in occupational health practice in Quebec, so it has forced the (overwhelmingly male) union health and safety committees to take a good look at health risks in women's jobs and, sometimes, to engage with the women's committees of their unions. These contacts have reinforced the women's committees and helped them diminish risks in women's jobs. The fact that the public health services were involved in identifying conditions that endangered pregnant women got doctors interested in women's working conditions, many of which were (surprise!) very unhealthy for all people exposed to them.[3] Most important, over time, the many attacks from employers were effective in stimulating strong alliances among unions, women's groups, feminist researchers, and public health professionals that have maintained the protections for pregnant women and extended to protections for other groups of women workers.[4]

I'm not the only one who seriously underestimated the difficulties in women's jobs and the dangers they pose for women's health. Employers, tribunals, and even co-workers can be as obtuse as I was. But listening to union women inspired me to learn about ergonomic analysis, an ideal tool for revealing hidden hazards.

What is ergonomic analysis?

Alain Wisner and the others who founded the French approach to ergonomics thought that "ignorance" might be what kept employers from providing a healthy workplace, and that science could perhaps fix this. Work was to be analyzed scientifically, using the acquired knowledge to transform the work process and environment so as to protect workers' health without hurting productivity.

At the core of the analysis was patient, long-term observation of the work and exchanges with the workers so the ergonomist could understand the constraints and imperatives behind each action.[5] Why does the sewing machine operator raise her shoulder in an awkward position? Ergonomists start from the premise that she isn't too dumb to notice that her shoulder is being hurt or too "resistant to change" to move her machine. So is it because her chair can't be adjusted? Because the piece of cloth is too big? Because her workbench is too wide? Because her supervisor has decided that is the one right way to perform that operation? Because sometimes she needs to be able to reach over to her colleague's machine to help her out?

Ergonomists may have ideas and theories about what is wrong, but we're not allowed to make them up all by ourselves. We need to validate our ideas with people actually doing the job. No, the women tell us, the problem isn't the chair; the chair is fine, it's that we have to rush so much. We don't have time to move it to the right position. And what would be the right position? How can we get the chair to stay in the right position, or support the shoulder, or lengthen the time available, or do away entirely with the operation that requires raising the shoulder? Back to the workplace for more observations and conversations with the workers. Repeat as necessary.

A key idea is that the aim of the ergonomic intervention is to enlarge workers' "operational leeway," or wiggle room, to enable them to protect their health while doing their jobs.[6] Workers will naturally adapt job parameters to their own capacities and needs if they have the leeway to do so. So making a chair height easily adjustable, providing a variety of tool sizes, and facilitating communication among workers are some ways of expanding operational leeway.

Only when ergonomists have thoroughly observed the work and considered the points of view of all the workplace participants, validating them in turn by further observations, can we make recommendations. And I was specifically taught that our recommendations could never be to eliminate certain workers or to apply pre-employment testing—the work had to be adapted to all workers, and not the other way around.

Ergonomists are not supposed to impose solutions. We must discuss our proposals for change with people in the workplace and, optimally, test them before putting them definitively in place. So ergonomic interventions have potential for the kind of empowerment feminists are interested in. The workers are partners in the attempts to understand work and they participate in making it better.[7]

Can feminist principles be applied to ergonomic interventions?

Catherine Cailloux-Teiger, one of the few women in the original band of French ergonomists, has pointed out that their very first formal ergonomic intervention, and most of those that followed, involved women workers and improved women's work.[8] Why did they study so many women's jobs? Probably because the risks in women's jobs tend to be less visible, so ergonomic analysis was necessary in order to reveal them. This invisibility is the flip side of men's assignment to visibly dangerous jobs. When work is obviously heavy, scary, or complicated, employers have tended to hire men; baggage handlers, soldiers, and mechanics are recruited primarily among men, and no one is surprised that they get backaches, bullet wounds, lead poisoning, and sore arms. But women's jobs tend to look easy, to require only "natural" abilities not considered to be skills, so Catherine's first ergonomics study was initiated just for that reason: women electronics workers were getting sick and having to leave the job, although it was classed as "light" work. Their male union representatives asked the scientists whether the women's problems were "really serious."

That initial study revealed many health risks on the electronics assembly line, such as prolonged standing in a static position, an extremely fast work pace, eyes fixed on small objects, and precise, fine movements with cramped hands . The ergonomists were able to propose some changes in the way the work stations were organized, but, especially, they were able to show that the women's health problems were not due to "nervous tension," but to the real working conditions. The ergonomists kept on studying women's jobs, and their interventions among telephone operators, administrative clerks, and sewing machine operators became classics in the field.[9]

However, in the ergonomics literature and in my classes, the gender of these workers was hidden behind the name "operators," or *opérateurs,* in the masculine gender.[10] I never knew that the textbook interventions I studied in Paris dealt with women workers. And, not only that, I was explicitly told not to think about gender. In my very first class at the Conservatoire national des arts et métiers, the professor asked all of us to describe our attempts to find a place to do our supervised internship. I said I had just arrived from Canada and didn't have any leads, but I wanted to study women's work, could anyone suggest a place? The professor replied curtly that there was no such thing as women's work, there was only work, which could and should be adapted to all populations.

Cailloux-Teiger suggests that one reason why ergonomists are reluctant to identify women in their interventions is that they fear that any mention of difficulties of women's work would provoke discriminatory practices—women might no longer be hired. And in fact my professor later told me he had wanted to avoid stereotyping.

But when I ignored him and studied older women cleaning toilets at a railway station, I found there was so such a thing as women's work, and it led to suffering. I had to name the task segregation. Women were specifically assigned to bending down and cleaning toilets, and men to driving water trucks, polishing handrails, and sweeping floors. The women's tasks involved a faster work speed, less help from machines, and more awkward postures. Not naming the discrimination would have left it invisible.

The same professor told us our interventions were to be "scientific," as opposed to "political." When I asked how he suggested handling differences between workers and management, or union-management disputes, he answered that ergonomists had to position themselves as neutral, slithering through cracks in the barriers between opposing groups and finding solutions acceptable to all. If significant risks to workers' health persisted and management balked at our suggestions, we couldn't do anything about this. When I pointed out that ergonomists were usually paid by management in the interests of reducing costs, my professor responded that we couldn't let that influence our stance; it had to be persistently "neutral" and promote health at the same time as job performance. Only a few ergonomists worked with unions at that time.

The scientific approach to demonstrating risks in women's work

Nicole Vézina has been my model, both intellectually and morally, since I first learned about ergonomics. Her approach to ergonomic analysis is thorough and profound. The first highly educated member of a working-class family, she really, really wants to improve workers' lives. Her way to do this is to identify aspects of work activity and work organization that damage workers and are not essential to the production process. In other words, she looks for environmental changes she can get employers to accept.

She started working out this approach during her MSc studies in the late 1970s. Supervised by Donna Mergler, Nicole's first study involved workers in nine poultry processing plants. With the help of the CSN union health and safety experts, Nicole and Donna talked to the workers and learned about their problems. They administered a detailed questionnaire about the workers' health problems and working environment.

The responses to the questionnaire revealed a number of work-related health problems, mostly pain from repetitive work, cuts from knives, viral warts, and menstrual problems from exposures to cold temperatures.[11] Nicole and Donna collaborated with the union to produce a graphics pamphlet called *Abattoir : Ne nous laissons pas abattre!* (Slaughterhouse: Let's Not Let Ourselves Be Slaughtered!), describing the workers' health and safety problems and suggesting solutions. The union-university collaboration succeeded in getting official recognition for the problems and in identifying viral warts as a disease that was specific to poultry workers, thus eligible for workers' compensation.[12] The unions also used the results to fix some problems with the collective agreement. Nicole then went to France for her PhD, learning to apply ergonomic analysis in the slaughterhouses there.

But Nicole did not stop at that. She is almost unbelievably focused. When she finds a problem, she learns all there is to know about it and she concentrates on fixing it, whatever it takes, for however long. In poultry processing, Nicole saw that her work had opened up a possibility for change. She had found that the workers were cutting themselves because their knives were too dull. They would try to cut, debone, and defat the chicken or turkey at the high speed of the assembly line, but the knives would slip and careen onto their hands and arms. Also, cutting up a bird every few seconds is really hard to do if your knife is dull, so the workers were pushing down too hard and having terrible, disabling aches and pains in their shoulders, arms, wrists, and hands.[13] The birds had to pass through workers' hands at the rate of one a minute, with no time for sharpening knives.

Even more important, a lot of workers didn't really know how to make a knife sharp. What was the right sharpener? Used at what angle? How thin should the knife edge be made? So, over the following decades, Nicole and her students got slaughterhouse workers to identify colleagues with knife-sharpening skills, consulted with professional knife sharpeners in the community, and described the principal movements involved in getting a knife sharp. They categorized, assessed, and optimized those movements. They then collaborated with workers and employers to make a video on knife sharpening that they used to train workers to be expert knife sharpeners.[14] Her video *Coupera ou coupera pas?* (Will It Cut?) was shown to slaughterhouse workers in Quebec and France. Her team carefully assessed the success of their training and worked to improve it.

An essential part of all this effort was that it involved minimum annoyance and expenditure for the employer, and even improved production. There were no open challenges to authority. Gender relations were never brought up explicitly, nor was there any other overt question of power relations. But Nicole quietly made sure that both women and men were included among the expert trainers, to make sure the training extended to both genders.

Nicole herself is well aware of gender issues. Already in her first study, Nicole had carefully characterized (and published) the division of tasks in poultry processing by gender (Figure 6.1). Men slaughtered the chickens, women and a few men eviscerated them and began cutting them up, women did the fine cleaning, taking off the last bits of extra fat, women and men packed the chicken parts, and men put them into freezers and shipped them.[15]

Figure 6.1 Division of labour by gender in a poultry processing plant in Quebec in the 1980s

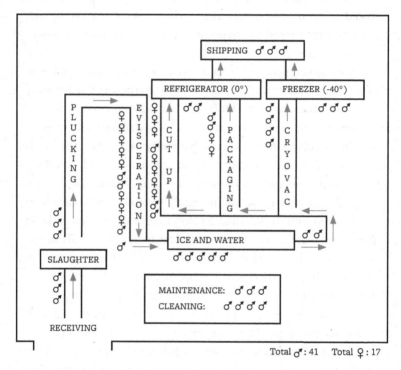

Source: Donna Mergler, Carole Brabant, Nicole Vézina, and Karen Messing, "The Weaker Sex?: Men in Women's Working Conditions Report Similar Health Symptoms," *Journal of Occupational Medicine* 29,5 (1987), 419.

In 1995, Nicole wrote one of the first careful descriptions of the physical aspects of the gender division of labour in factories.[16] She said the women's jobs on a turkey-processing line were "wearing" (*usant*) because they involved repeated movements, precision, and awkward postures resulting, over time, in localized pain. The men's jobs were called "limiting" (*limitant*) because they required the use of explosive physical strength at levels at the limit of men's capacities. Women reported pain more often but about the same number of work accidents as men, and many women's work accidents occurred when they replaced men at such tasks as cracking the chicken apart. So the occupational health problems were more visible at the men's jobs than the women's.

After Nicole finished her doctorate in ergonomics, she came home and applied for a professorship in our biology department. On the eve of the academic presentation on her thesis work that was to determine whether she would get the job, I gave her a pep talk about how she should have confidence in her abilities, she should just tell herself she was the best. She didn't go for that strategy. Instead, she said: "I'm going to visualize the women's faces, the women in the processing plants." I have learned over time that it is no use trying to make Nicole talk or think about her own interests; she is unable to separate herself from her solidarity with others and particularly with low-paid women workers. I remember the twinkle in her eye when she told me about how she had managed to inveigle women into the group of knife-sharpening trainers.

As a professor, Nicole has trained a series of intelligent students to do careful, thorough studies that avoid giving the hiccups to factory management, and women workers are undoubtedly better off for them. She avoids the kind of intensely emotional confrontation that we provoked in the hospitals, among the government health and safety organizations, and in union meetings. She tends to resolve any conflict between health and equality in favour of health, while giving a push to equality when she can.

With her students, she has carefully characterized the work of women who operate sewing machines, check out groceries, put boots together, and sort packages, among many other jobs. In each case, her idea is to defend the workers, give them more leeway, and reduce the workload.[17] She testified in favour of women postal workers claiming workers' compensation for shoulder pain, demonstrating that they coded fifteen to twenty packages per minute, moving an average of 12,000 kilograms per day with their left hands, although each package was relatively small.[18]

The fact that physical demands on women workers tend to be less visible than physical demands in men's jobs makes it possible for ergonomists to surprise management with their observations of the women's jobs. And Nicole has been able to highlight a more general problem for women in factories: women are concentrated toward the end of assembly lines, which means they are at the mercy of the speed of the men before them. So they have to correct whatever mistakes have been made earlier. By alerting management to this source of overload, Nicole and her students have helped to ease the pressure on many women workers.

Let's look at her efforts to popularize the sit/lean chair. As in many other jurisdictions, Quebec has legal language requiring employers to provide seats in the workplace, but, here as elsewhere, many low-paid service workers are forced to stand all day. Nicole was a pioneer in the struggle for seats for supermarket cashiers, bank tellers, and others who stand at work without moving, an exposure that is dangerous for the circulatory and musculoskeletal systems and is more common among women.[19] She documented the harm from standing, figured out that an adjustable sit/lean chair would be the best solution for cashiers, did research to find the very best seat to recommend, tried to influence the health and safety authorities to require seats, worked with supermarket owners to make them accept seats, and worked with unions to make them aware of the risks of prolonged standing. She spent at least ten years patiently sitting on government-industry committees, listening to the ever-evolving reasons offered by the employers as to why supermarket cashiers couldn't sit at work just yet.

Some of her efforts were successful. She testified for a union and helped win a seat for a supermarket worker with backache. One of her students became a labour inspector and imposed seats for workers in a credit union, resulting, in the long run, in seats for most bank tellers in Quebec. Another of her former students successfully testified in favour of seats for bookstore clerks in a major chain, facing down two appeals. And another CINBIOSE graduate testified for seats for casino workers, in a second successful case.[20] But, despite an enormous weight of evidence that seats are necessary, and labour standards that explicitly require seats to be provided, many, many service-sector workers are still standing without moving, with aching limbs, backs, and legs, risking cardiovascular damage.[21] And most of them are women.

Politics and ergonomics

Nicole's team has demonstrated scientifically that many jobs held by women hurt them, enabling some women to get compensation and transforming some jobs where the workers are women. But there has not been much change in social vision. When the Quebec government proposed changes in the health and safety laws in 2020, our research group calculated that 7 percent of women, compared to 22 percent of male workers, were considered to be at high risk and thus eligible for the most intense prevention efforts. Conversely, 72 percent of women and 53 percent of men were put in the category at lowest risk.

Women still don't have much political power in their factories or low-paid service jobs. So the women's committees and health and safety committees of the trade unions explicitly invited us, as their partners, to participate in social change. We were supposed not only to improve work, but to support organizational justice in the workplace. The next chapter will describe this partnership.

7.
LOOKING THE
DRAGON IN
THE FACE

was about forty-five when I decided to profit more from Quebec winters and brush up on my skiing. My lessons went okay until my instructor wanted me to go from stem (snowplow) turns to real parallel turns with my skis pointing downhill. My own aim was to avoid building up any speed at all, so I ended each turn with my skis pointing up the hill, unable to continue smoothly. "You have to look the dragon in the face!" yelled my instructor, wanting me to face down the hill. And I did, and it worked, and I have been skiing the expert trails for over thirty years.

Looking the dragon in the face has generally been my ergonomics team's approach to intervention in women's work. Sexism in the workplace is a pretty big, flame-spouting dragon, and our open interest in gender equality and promoting the health of women workers has gotten us into trouble with employers, granting agencies, and even a few unions. For many years some granting agencies explicitly blocked our access to funds to study women's occupational health. The head of a major research organization specified to its communications department that any mention of women's work had to exclude our research results or attribute them to other researchers. When I was invited to speak at the offices of the work-ers' compensation commission on International Women's Day, the department heads got a memo saying they should discourage their workers from attending. (What do you know—that memo got me a full lecture hall.)

Our research alliance with the union women's committees meant that we couldn't hide our interest in gender from employers or workers, even if we wanted to. Not for us the subtle balancing of forces and quiet negotiations taught by Nicole and our professors in France. Our work has fed into union actions and even led to strikes. We were only allowed into the workplace for observations where the union was able to get us in—where contract language provided for union expertise, where employers and unions agreed there was a problem, or where the women's issues initially appeared harmless to the employer.

Our approach to prolonged standing has been explicitly political. We put pressure on a deputy minister so a question on prolonged standing at work was added, at the last minute, to a Quebec public health survey, and our colleagues in public health have kept up the pressure so that the question is included whenever the province asks about occupational health.[1] We have worked with the public health experts to analyze the data and communicated the results to scientists and unions.[2] We have used the data pedagogi-cally to show that analyzing data on prolonged standing separately for women and men revealed risks for both sexes (see chapter 12).[3] We have presented the data internationally and found allies among researchers in Canada and other countries who joined with us to produce data nuancing the prevailing theory that "sitting is the new smoking." It has been the accumulation of many people's research and strong union actions that has won seats for store clerks in Quebec and California.[4]

Our CINBIOSE research team, led by Marie Laberge, recently

got a grant to examine the question of whether incorporating sex and gender in health interventions really improves Canadians' health. But we need to ask, what kinds of interventions? Can the conflict between health and gender equality really be resolved? What approaches work the best? What are the obstacles? What helps?

L'Invisible qui fait mal—a research partnership

In the 1990s, the Quebec health ministry established a program to promote community-scientist alliances to improve health, and our union-researcher partnership squeezed its way into the definition of a community health partnership. From 1993 to my retirement in 2008, we got a series of generous grants to observe women's work: cleaners, bank tellers, elementary and secondary school teachers, adult education teachers, communications technicians, health care aides, food servers, telephone operators, trade school teachers, hotel workers, retail workers, special education aides, teleworkers, and hospital receptionists, among others.

In each case, we had help from our university outreach service, which set up joint committees to guide the research process. The committees included people from the union women's committees and from the local unions involved. When the women's committees picked good, active unions, which they almost always did, the process was exciting—we had to answer tough questions and we got stimulating feedback. The whole scientific process was interactive and everyone came out a lot smarter. And—big bonus for us—we heard about developing workplace problems well before the scientific competition. Precarious work schedules became a thing in the literature in the 2000s; we heard about it from the unions in 1993.

But even while we partnered with the women's committees, we

couldn't always focus directly on gender during our interventions. In our first series of investigations in 1993–95, the unions asked us to look at women's most common jobs, like receptionist, bank teller, and elementary school teacher. Since there were almost no men in these jobs, gendered task assignments and gender relations did not figure in our work activity descriptions. Although union members did occasionally bring up examples of discrimination, we put most of our energy into describing the invisible risks in these jobs and suggesting improvements, just as my ergonomics professors had taught me. We documented the long hours bank tellers spent on their feet, how the teachers coped with the growing number of children with behaviour issues, how hospital receptionists dealt with patients who had cognitive problems or who spoke neither English nor French. We proposed appropriate seats for the tellers,[5] smaller class sizes for the teachers,[6] and adapted telephone headsets for the receptionists.[7] Nicole was officially a member of the partnership and her input into our studies was invaluable. The unions could use our scientific results to produce concrete changes in their local working conditions. Aggregated, they also showed that women's work involves hidden risks, so our law professor colleagues and the union women's committees could also use them to promote more general recognition of women's occupational health problems.[8]

Our next wave of studies involved women performing tasks previously assigned to men, like those I have described in chapters 1, 2, and 3. Many women had come into those jobs through legal action by women's groups or unions, so gender was salient for the employer, even an irritant. We had more difficulty changing those jobs because many women were not happy about being singled out. The women often tried to look as much like the men as possible, resisting any suggestion that their bodies, their work techniques, or their abilities were different from those of their colleagues. They had been quietly putting up with psychological harassment and even physical violence to make their way in an alien system, and they didn't want us to make them stand out.

These were the studies that made us think about biology, sex, and gender in the most practical terms. Why was Rose having difficulty lifting patients? What kind of tool belt did Suzanne need? These studies also made the unions work the hardest to assimilate the results. In fact, it took years after these interventions for the results to percolate through the union structures into policy and practice. Through a union-sponsored course in women's occupational health, a push for more women in construction jobs, new legislation on harassment, or just open discussions about the gendered distribution of work, we could slowly see our partnership hadn't totally wasted everyone's time.

Gender, work, and family

In the early 2000s, attacks on women's jobs in the service sector intensified. Opening hours expanded and work times became irregular and unpredictable. Employers treated workers as interchangeable units that could be slotted into service use patterns,[9] and started aligning work schedules more closely with microvariations in demand over minutes and hours. Workers had to juggle wildly to reconcile their schedules with their home responsibilities.

So we had to think about sex and gender, both. When we thought about work schedules, we had to think about the association of night work with breast cancer (sex) and work-family balance (gender). And we had to fight the tendency to stereotype women at the same time. Yes, women are in danger of breast cancer from night work, but men's physiology suffers from night work as well. Yes, domestic responsibilities should be shared, and it is not a good idea to base policy on a presumption that only women do child care and elder care. But workplace law and policy were designed at a time when the (male) workers could rely on a woman at home to take care of domestic issues. So that now, work processes interfere in many different ways with how family life is organized. And those people who do the organizing are mostly women.

The unions in our partnership told us that schedule issues mobilize women. Low-paid women workers need to have enough paid hours to survive this week and they need the hours to be compatible with their children's schedules, starting now. They don't want their employer mad at them and they need their supervisors to feel friendly and well-disposed to accommodate their needs. They put a lot more energy into schedule negotiations than into trying to get seats at work, for example.

Our partnership undertook a series of studies of work schedules that showed us how domestic and paid work activities intertwine.

Work and home

Our first study, in the late 1990s, opened my eyes to one way work demands were invading domestic life.[10] Call centre workers, almost all women, had little control over their working hours and were scheduled with dizzying irregularity. Since anticipated call volume per fifteen-minute period could be related to the weather, holidays, and television offerings, their scheduled eight-hour shifts could start at any time from 6 a.m. to 4 p.m., change on successive days, and vary from one week to the next. There were new schedule assignments every two weeks, with three or four days' notice. All this in the interest of making sure there wasn't a single extra telephone operator at work for any fifteen-minute period.

While the call centre optimized its staffing, the domestic sphere was pushed into chaos. Women could schedule nothing in advance—family doctors' appointments, meetings with the teacher, birthday parties fell victim to the employers' needs. Both women and men complained that they couldn't schedule romantic dinners, sign up for evening classes, or play on sports teams. Children's homework could be supervised (or not) by as many as eight different people over a two-week period. Since the workers we studied were members of what had been a very strong, militant union, they were tied to their jobs by accumulated seniority and relatively good salaries, even as their schedules became impossible.

The union was able to negotiate our way in to do a few hours of observations, so we could see that the women were stuck in their assigned seats, forbidden to move, to talk to each other, or to make or receive personal calls. We watched as the women walked up to the boards where their schedules were posted, and listened to their reactions. The mothers among them used a wide array of cumbersome strategies when they found they wouldn't be able to make an assigned shift—requesting changes from their unwilling supervisors, posting their need to trade shifts on a bulletin board, multiple babysitters, live-in relatives—but nothing worked for long. I smelled desperation, even heard about a suicide, but could come up with few useful suggestions. The employer was impervious to any ideas about making the schedules more predictable. Our only accomplishment was to make some supervisors aware that women who had trouble arriving on time for work were less often "irresponsible" than overwhelmed. And telling some scientists and policymakers that atypical schedules had tremendous social costs. Over time, with our colleagues in law, the unions were able to push for some better social policies like advance notice for schedule changes.

Our second study of work scheduling pointed out the importance of stable teams for health care. Ana Maria Seifert showed that when nurses in a Quebec hospital were assigned to work anywhere it suited the employer, patient care suffered from a lack of continuity.[11] The chance of a patient seeing the same nurse two days in a row was less than 50 percent, meaning not only that the patient lost out on care, but that the nurses had to take extra time to catch up on recent developments in the patients' health. In addition, communication among nurses was hampered by the constant shuttling. Of eleven different schedule pairings during a one-week period, only two of the teams worked together twice in a row. So the nurses' efficiency was affected as well as their sense of meaning in their work. During the pandemic, the shuffling of health care workers from place to place and the instability of work teams became a lethal source of infection for both workers and patients.

If our first study about work and family educated us about intrusive schedules, and our second about team disruption, our third made us realize how manager attitudes can affect the work/home interface. This third study involved a publicly funded seniors' residence whose director fancied himself a philosopher. He was delighted to have university researchers come to study and presumably admire his perfectly run establishment. Instead we observed an exhausted 100 percent female workforce trying to survive in a rats' nest of backbiting and competition for decent schedules.[12] The philosopher relied on two overworked, underresourced female schedule managers to resolve all problems, heaping blame on them if the workers complained about their schedules.

The schedules had to cover twenty-four hours a day, seven days a week, and shifts were assigned by seniority. But management was reluctant to commit to hiring regular staff, so they assigned lots of shifts to on-call workers at the last minute. The schedule managers would call in the health care aides in order of seniority until they succeeded in filling an assignment. They used a lot of ingenuity to improvise scheduling software that would enable them to follow and adjudicate the myriad requests for schedule adjustments and changes, but the director gave them no logistic or moral support. There was no policy support either—the schedule managers had to decide to accept or reject requests for schedule changes based on whether they believed an individual worker and thought she was trying hard to come in on time, leaving themselves open to accusations of favouritism. Meanwhile, the workers had learned how to survive—by impressing the schedule managers, by making as few commitments as possible in advance, by myriad invisible arrangements with friends and family. Workers were not allowed to use their cell phones on the job, but of course they communicated with husbands, babysitters, grandmothers, and schools—it just took more time because they had to hide. A mess.

We learned from this study how banal occurrences become disasters when workers are rigidly scheduled—a snowstorm, car trouble, illness, parking problems, a son getting into trouble, a daughter unexpectedly qualifying for a championship athletic contest, a husband called away. The union used our report to negotiate some changes in the collective agreement and to press for a daycare in some unused space at the residence. As far as we could tell, the philosopher learned nothing from our report. He used our presentation to attack his poor old schedule managers yet again, despite our protests.

I heard from him again in 2020, when the disastrous effects of shuffling workers around were made manifest in the epidemic of COVID-19 among health care workers. My colleagues and I wrote a letter to the newspapers suggesting workers should be assigned to regular schedules and specific areas, so they could enjoy long-term relationships with their patients, be safer, and have more regular lives.[13] In response, he sent me pages of theory which, I have to say, I didn't understand. And no one else from the health services responded to our letter, although several union leaders wrote to support our suggestions.

In fact, as long ago as 2011, our union friends had come up with what looked like the perfect place to influence schedules, with true employer collaboration for the first time. A large retail employer was worried about its huge employee turnover, over 100 percent per year—meaning that most employees lasted only a few months. The stores really wanted to be told how to improve employee satisfaction, and we were delighted to accept the task. The union lost no time in introducing us to the vice president in charge of human resources. We would figure out how to improve the process of schedule selection and make both employees and employer happy.

We had no problem diagnosing what was wrong or in producing documentation through observations and a questionnaire.[14] The scheduling process was rigid, arbitrary, and unreasonable. Most of the schedules included periods when daycare centres were closed[15]—early morning, evenings, and weekends. Schedules varied unpredictably, with shift start times varying from 6 a.m. to 6 p.m. for the same person over the same week. Workers got their schedules Thursday or Friday for the week starting Sunday—two or three days' notice. No one could be reached at work in case of emergency. Since workers had a hard time coping, they often called at the last minute to say they couldn't make their shifts, forcing the department manager to call in other workers or to pressure those at work to stay on. Since the managers had to cover the shifts themselves if they couldn't find a replacement, they could get angry. Missing too many shifts or refusing to help a manager could result in bad shifts in the future.

Only about a third of workers reported any family responsibilities, compared with about 45 percent of the working-age population at large,[16] indicating that people with families might be avoiding these jobs or leaving them. About the same proportion of workers

(33 percent) said they had a lot of difficulty reconciling their work schedule with their personal lives. And we had no trouble identifying gender issues. Women, especially those with family responsibilities, had much more difficulty with schedules and with the work-family interface. The women with families generally wanted to work fewer hours than did the women without families, while the opposite held true for the men, leading us to believe that the women saw their primary family responsibility as care while the men with families felt more pressure to make money.

Women were usually cashiers, and their jobs were physically demanding because they worked standing and they had to handle heavy packages. They were often scheduled at the last minute, and interactions with customers could be stressful. The men's jobs involved physical strength or recognized technical skills—unlike the less visible tact, humour, and patience required at the cash register—so the men were paid more and it was they whom the employer said they wanted to retain. The employer felt we were insufficiently interested in the "qualified" (i.e., male) workforce and too interested in work-family interactions. A vice president told us he didn't want to hear any more, ever, about work-family balancing, although he had known of our interest from the start. Management eventually booted us out, refusing to show our report to their employees. In a particularly nefarious move, they offered to send our report privately to those employees we would identify as being particularly interested in the results, but we didn't like the idea of informing on "disloyal" employees and refused.

This particular union was cowed by management, so the participants never saw the results—a first (and last) in my career as a researcher. The union didn't seem to be very interested in our report overall. The study's only positive result was to inspire a single store to create a few more stable jobs with predictable schedules. We were disappointed not to be able to help more.

But the study did result in a big piece of luck for us. One of our best research assistants was a master's student in communication studies, Mélanie Lefrançois.[17] I swooped down and induced her to do a PhD in ergonomics and communication, jointly supervised with a colleague in the Communications Department, Johanne Saint-Charles. At that time, our union friends were asking us to do another work-family study and Mélanie, mother of two pre-adolescents, was interested. The women's committee representative took us to a regional union meeting where we asked whether anyone was interested in a work-family intervention. Maurice Arseneault, from a transport union, was the most convincing, and he took us back to meet his members. He wanted us to look into the work schedules in his company, which I'll call Transpeq. It was the first time I had to work closely with a big, male-dominated union.

We started with the group of cleaners, 36 percent women. Maurice helped Mélanie meet all the key people. It turns out that training in communications comes in very handy when setting up an ergonomic intervention with a hostile employer. Mélanie, who has a beautiful smile, quickly figured out which managers and union officials needed to be onside, organized meetings with them, got their approval for the project, and started observations. She felt she needed to get trained as a cleaner and spent some time working on cleaning teams to get to know the job before starting the ergonomic observations. She pretty much lived in the workplace for a year and got to know all the workers and managers. They loved her.

The job she studied was not easy. Cleaning the tight spaces on the transport equipment involved lots of awkward postures, time pressure, coordinated teamwork, and uncomfortable, hot conditions, especially in summer. The work teams were together day after day, providing support and even helping out if someone wasn't feeling well or needed to deal with a situation at home. But there could be tensions, too—we heard racist and sexist remarks that made us cringe. Some women said they had felt threatened by certain men, especially late in the evening.

We spent a lot of time observing the actual scheduling process. It was more humane than in retail or at the call centre. Every six months the company posted the hundreds of different shifts it was offering and workers picked theirs in order of seniority, with the help of the union rep. But choosing a schedule was no easy task. You needed to make a number of complicated choices: a time of day, a sequence of days on / days off, a work team, and a type of equipment to clean. Or else you could decide to be on call for a variety of shifts. Each choice had consequences. The period (day? evening? night?) determined workload and fatigue as well as pay rate. Time of day also affected commuting time, including whether you could find a parking space anywhere near the job. The sequence of days on/ off could be 5/2, 4/2, 4/3, 4/4, or on call (replacements), determining hours per day as well as how many weekends you had to work and how tired you would be by the time your days off rolled around.

> "I sleep three hours a day, and my schedules are hard with my new boyfriend. I'm always running around for babysitters, my mom helps the best she can. And my daughters need to go to the doctor often . . . so I'm late, I miss work . . ." (female cleaner)

The longer you were on the job, the more things you knew you had to think about when you picked your schedule. Some types of equipment were easier to clean, or easier for smaller people, or required bigger work teams. And a congenial work team turned out to be vitally necessary for a whole bunch of reasons. If you came in with low energy or in a bad mood, would the others cover for you? If you were tired or upset, would your mates be supportive or critical?

Would they be fair in sharing out the cleaning tasks or would one person (the Arab, the African, the woman) always end up doing the toilets? Did everyone clean to the same standard?

And, for the even more sophisticated, there were additional things to think about. If I take this schedule and my friend takes that schedule, we will be able to swap sometimes to get an occasional extra day off in exchange for doing a double shift—if I'm not too tired to do a double, that is. If my very senior friend with the nice day shift whispers to me that she will be going on maternity leave in July, it is worth it for me to opt for on call for the chance of grabbing her wonderful hours in a few weeks' time, at the risk of being plugged into horrible slots before she goes on leave? What if she has a miscarriage?

And what about people who had less access to information, like new hires, minorities, immigrants, and people who didn't speak English or French? They didn't know how to choose their schedules and they didn't hear about all the possibilities to work the system.

Once workers had been around for several years, they could figure out the implications of the proposed schedules fairly rapidly and pick their schedules intelligently. But sometimes the company would throw a wrench in the works. Like the year they decreed that most of the part-time workers would work five days on / two days off. A disaster, because any schedule based on a regular seven-day period (as opposed to 4/2 or 4/4) means that the few lucky, very senior workers who can grab Monday to Friday on / Saturday and Sunday off will get every single weekend off, but that more than half the workers will have no weekend days off at all for the next six months.

Or the time the company overlapped shifts, on purpose, so that exchanges became difficult to impossible. Even after we explained the importance of flexibility to the employer representative (who didn't look as if he was listening), they refused to change it. Events like this explained why the bulletin board where the company posted the schedules was called the "wailing wall."

Mélanie and I installed ourselves next to the wailing wall during the schedule bids and talked to the workers about the choices they were making. We learned that they put a lot of energy into getting with the right work team. This choice had very practical implications, given the physical and emotional requirements of the job.

> "When there's a heat wave and we've been running all day,
> non-stop, no water, no break, someone will brush your arm
> and it will turn into a big fight." (male cleaner)

Choosing the work team, a team leader, the hours worked, and the days off were the major considerations, but we also heard about women not wanting shifts at the same time as scary male co-workers and about complex gaming around on-call assignments.

The union was very involved in helping workers choose schedules. It had some input in negotiating the schedule and it provided expert advice during the whole period of schedule choice. But although its actual power to influence the schedule was quite limited, workers would end up blaming the union representatives when they were unable to rectify unfair situations (notably, the overlapping schedules). At other times, worker solidarity was amazing, for instance when a band of senior workers decided that they would leave a day shift open for a mother exhausted from working night shifts. Although the opposite could also happen: some people knowingly chose schedules that were good for them but that "bumped" those next in line off their usual work team. This was not necessarily a winning strategy: the teams, furious at losing a valued less-senior member, could make the intruder's life miserable for the next six months.

A lot of cleaners had hard lives to start with. Many were immigrants with limited French who had to struggle every day just to get themselves to the jobsite on time. Some were people of colour who had to put up with the most horrible of the racist epithets; it was heartbreaking to watch them try to smile, and we were tempted to leave our "observer" posture to intervene.

The scheduling problems rendered their lives even harder. Some divorced men with one week on / one week off custody had to deal with child-care challenges. But the most extreme scheduling problems we saw involved women workers. The night shift was composed, amazingly, of mothers who chose that shift because there was little competition for it and it left their days "free" for family-related activities. One single mother made us cry with her stories of dealing with the schedule, the work team, and her son's numerous medical appointments.[18]

> "Last year I thought I was going to catch a cancer or something, I was going to get sick, I was going to die." (cleaner, mother of a chronically sick child)

Mélanie made an important observation during this study that has been critical to our understanding. She found that schedules were not the only way that the work put pressure on domestic life—professional and personal lives were closely bound together in many other ways. First, there was fatigue management. The work was heavy and cleaners got hot and uncomfortable. They had to arrange their work life so they wouldn't go home exhausted and grumpy and be impatient with their families. They needed to be nice to the other services that conditioned their break times, so they wouldn't get their breaks at the beginning or the very end of their shifts. Similarly, they needed to develop supportive social lives at work, since they might need to be covered if child-care arrangements collapsed or a home crisis made them late for work. They were also dependent on teammates and other colleagues to get information and tips on scheduling. So they put a lot of energy into choosing their work teams and building those relationships.[19]

And they also needed to set up just the right amount of benevolence from their supervisors. Too much "brown-nosing," and they would lose respect and support from co-workers. Too few favours for management, and they would lose any leeway they might have accessed to get leave if a child was ill or to get information useful for choosing a work schedule. Mélanie's combined expertise in communications and ergonomics helped us see that building and facilitating teamwork are critical for managing work-family interactions.

When the dragon is hiding

Gender almost never came up explicitly during this study. The union always spoke about work-family conflict in general. But gender (as well as ethnicity and language) was embedded in the choices of work teams, in avoiding certain potential teammates, in how the supervisors viewed the workers' family-related problems with the schedule. I had the impression that a lot of the women's energy in this male-dominated workplace was devoted to keeping their family problems invisible at work, while the men may have felt freer to bring them up. In fact, when the union executive told us about formal grievances they were dealing with in relation to work-family conflict, the cases had all been brought by men.

We made forty-eight suggestions to union and management, and the union people say they have been very useful. We recommended measures to increase respect for cleaners, to get better tools, to distribute the workload more fairly. We strongly suggested that managers develop policy to facilitate the work-family interface and to combat racism. We also questioned the allocation of certain tasks according to gender, and we proposed the formation of a women's committee. For the first time ever, the union used its power to block the schedule proposed by management.

Mélanie's expertise in communication also led us to develop an instrument for people to help them choose their schedules—a pamphlet explaining some of the things they needed to know when making their choices. The union loved it and asked for it to be adapted for their other workers in the other, 99 percent male sections of Transpeq whose work schedules were equally complicated and distressing.

But, aside from some remarks about sexual, sexist (and racist) harassment, we didn't see anywhere we could legitimately talk about gender in the report. So if it is not naturally part of the union discussions about the work-family interface, where does gender come up? Where was the dragon's face? Should we have made gender more explicit? How? And how could our interventions have worked better to promote equality as well as better schedules?

As with our earlier studies, one problem has to do with statistics (see also chapter 12). Statistical analysis requires that you examine the factors you are interested in (gender and schedules) while controlling for all the other things that vary. When you examine workplace health, many workplace parameters are common to all of the workers in a department—they breathe the same air, have the same management, have similar task assignments. But when you look at the work-family interface, there is a lot more variability. We talked to and/or observed about a hundred cleaning workers, and they had very different family situations. They dealt with the whole range of work-family challenges—a wife in another province, one week on / one week off custody arrangements, single parenting, a husband who travelled for work, night courses, a long commuting distance, a sick grandmother who had cut back on babysitting.

We didn't have enough people in our workplace to be able to do complicated statistical analysis looking at gender in all the different situations (not to mention age, seniority, language, immigrant status, and ethnicity).

So we had no evidence that could demonstrate to everyone in that workplace that women needed any special consideration. Was it necessary? Or should we have tried harder to help develop solidarity and support among women workers? But the women had already done that for themselves, on their teams and with their friends.

Certainly, Mélanie's presence in the workplace was a comfort and help to the women who talked to her about their child-care problems and their fears of certain colleagues. And the Transpeq union now has a women's committee, in part due to nagging from our team. But could we have done more to help women access the solidarity normally available through the union?

Is the personal really political?
Is the political very personal?

When I was a young feminist in the 1960s, everyone was quoting the phrase "the personal is political." No one seems to know who said it first or where, but what we meant was that the most intimate relationships take place in a sociopolitical context. We excitedly applied feminist analysis to every aspect of life, including each other's preferred sexual acts, desire to have children, taste in music and, of course, division of household tasks. Now our research group is having to think about that phrase fifty years later as we try to figure out how to apply work analysis to make paid work compatible with family responsibilities. Why is it so hard to apply gender analysis to action for work-family balancing?

As we discuss our successes and failures with others at the

university, we hear stories about what happens when gender comes up during research. As, for example, when one of my colleagues was presenting a request for research funds to a committee of employers, unions, and scientists. She mentioned gender toward the end of a list of potential impacts of the research—women trainers who used the research results might be able to gain more influence in jobs where men were the vast majority of workers. The outcry was such that the funder suggested they remove the offending word "women" from their list of potential outcomes. My colleague was surprised at the intensity of the feelings and at the fact that both women and men reacted negatively.

I have often seen counterproductive discussions of gender in unions, as well. I was at a large regional union meeting when Jessica Riel presented her MSc study of the work activity of high school teachers. Her observations revealed differences between women and men in time spent on various activities (women were more involved in discipline). The discussion rapidly degenerated into criticism of the other sex. Women were too fussy about discipline, they should learn to relax. No, men should take the rules more seriously, being lax just passed the problems on to other teachers. But if women would just maintain a friendly, supportive atmosphere, they would be more respected. No, women needed to maintain discipline, otherwise the boys in the class would feel entitled to act up . . . and so on, and so on. I have to say that the discussion didn't seem particularly fruitful. And the same thing happened in a different union confederation, where we started the meeting by presenting how workplace interventions could facilitate work-family balancing. Men then lined up at the microphones to explain that they did the dishes at home or that their wives were just better at doing laundry than they were.

Is this because we have not found the right way to moderate the discussion? Or is it that people's ideas and feelings about gender go very deep, and productive discussions would have to last a lot longer than unions can afford to free up workers from their jobs? Local union leadership changes often and different leaders have different interests, usually closely aligned with immediate pay and leave issues. And the fact that we have not found any employers interested in gender equality has made it difficult to do the kind of sustained long-term interventions that just might produce local change.

No question—the concepts of sex and gender carry an enormous emotional weight, and we have to struggle against the impulse to forget about them and concentrate on other aspects of work. At this writing, we have not found the right way to introduce gender considerations in the workplaces we have studied, even into discussions of work-family balancing. Given the limited time we spend in each workplace and our cultural distance from workers, maybe we just can't play a role in combatting this kind of inequality.

Such discussions require a lot of time and skilled orientation, and workplace-based women's committees are the ideal way to carry them forward, if we could find women who have the time and confidence to take on the responsibility of organizing discussions and dealing with the ensuing conflicts. In our own university women's committee—a near-ideal situation where the employer was in principle open to equality and diversity and the members were accustomed to complex discussions—our experience was not always easy. I think we will have to do more toward developing and encouraging change agents and encouraging our women's committees. We need to put developing solidarity at the forefront of our interventions.

Going higher up

In France, when Florence Chappert faced the employer's refusal to act on the injustice to women at the print shop (see chapter 4), she bumped her efforts up to the national policy level. With support from her government agency, she helped to pass a law that requires employers to examine and report workplace health and safety problems by gender, and to consider gender in their evaluation of workers' exposures.[20] Some French unions are gradually getting involved in making the law work, while Florence and her colleagues are now training employers to recognize and combat sexism.

Our Quebec unions suggested we also work with a group of law professors so that our research results could be translated into law and policy. What a good idea that turned out to be! Collaborating with the unions' legal specialists and health and safety services, the law professors examined gender in relation to questions like the fairness of compensation decisions involving women versus men, as well as policy surrounding workplace mental health, harassment, work-family interactions, precarious work, invasive work schedules, and globalization.[21] The ergonomists and law professors learned from each other's research, and together we felt we made good suggestions for workplace and policy change.[22] In Chile, after doing a study with our legal scholars and ergonomists, a group of feminist health advocates (Centro de los estudios de la mujer) collaborated with the public health authorities and with our former students Pamela Astudillo and Carlos Ibarra to make women's occupational health a subject of government concern as well as a union demand.[23] And we ourselves have been involved in a few court cases that required employers to adapt their workplaces for women.[24]

In Quebec, our colleagues in law and our union partners have used our research results to produce changes in the way our province considers work-family interactions and workplace sexual harassment, to support protection for pregnant women, to desegregate jobs, to require seats for store personnel and to promote consideration of women in occupational health and safety research. We have contributed to union discussions of policy. In fact, the union women's committees tell us that the mere fact that our partnership unites the women's committees with the traditionally male-dominated health and safety committees has given them new opportunities to influence union practices. In other words, our research has been effective because it fed into solidarity at the union confederation level.

Same genders, different genders?

In chapters 4 and 5, I showed why I think that treating women and men as if they have the same bodies ends up feeding into inequality at work and can cause health problems for women. But I also showed that emphasizing male-female biological differences can contribute to exaggerating the differences and encourage stereotyping. Feminists need to walk a fine line between recognizing sex differences and overemphasizing them.

I think the same is true of gender differences. We think of social roles as more fluid than biology, and they are, but they are pretty hard to escape. We see this especially when we try to make workplaces more family-friendly. Despite all the men who really try to be good fathers and share household tasks, most of the burden of work-family balancing still falls on women, and it is usually women who are blamed and who blame ourselves when something goes wrong. And despite all the talk about workplace equality, men usually feel more pressure to bring in a regular salary. So discussing work-family issues in the workplace falls into some of the same traps as discussing sex differences: Should we mention gender, at the risk of feeding into gender stereotypes? Should we ignore the fact that work-family interference disproportionately hurts women at work?

The most obvious example of a gender puzzle is the use of seniority in determining work schedules, in many non-unionized workplaces as well as unions. I should start by saying that almost everyone, workers and managers, likes using seniority to establish priorities because it is a better system than letting the managers decide all by themselves and then be accused of favouritism. However—the average male worker is more senior than the average woman, and the average older worker is more senior than the average younger person. So women with young children are among those with the greatest need but the least entitlement to family-friendly shifts and vacation times.

Just the gender aspects of the seniority question can lead to headaches. Should people with young children get some kind of priority for shifts and holidays? But what if they are men with young children and their wives don't do paid work? What if they are women whose husbands work at home? What about women who care for an aging parent? Or men with aging parents—how would we know if the men's mom and sisters were doing all the caring?

Would we want gender roles to be explicitly mentioned in seniority rules? Wouldn't that block career paths for all women? And what about gender-fluid people with children?

So on the one hand, denying that most domestic responsibilities fall on women can lead to suffering, while planning policy as if women were the only caregivers would strike a terrible blow to gender equality. The only solution would seem to be to adapt the workplace so that it interferes as little as possible with family life, by regularizing shifts, facilitating shift exchanges, minimizing night and weekend work, and facilitating child and elder care. And, more broadly, by making work less exhausting.[25] But I have not seen a lot of employers racing to be the most family-friendly workplace.

It's a big dragon

We have not been able to kill the dragon, but we have become aware of its enormous size and put a little water on the flames from its mouth. The combination of ergonomics with legal expertise has been helpful in carrying our local research findings into the policy arena. We hope Simone de Beauvoir's ghost will be happy that we have gotten some recognition for the problems of the "second sex" and the "second gender" at work.[26] We and our friends the legal scholars have helped the unions make progress on humanizing work schedules.[27]

We didn't do much to improve the lives of women in non-traditional jobs, but we probably helped the union women's committees in pushing for change and in their own struggle for survival. And those committees are soldiering on, fostering discussions of gender in the unions. In Quebec, women's rates of unionization have climbed steadily, while the numbers of unionized men are slowly declining. The fact that jobs are becoming more precarious and work hours more invasive is making work-family issues more of a union priority. We hope the unions will survive in the current unfriendly climate.

What have we learned about intervening in workplaces where equality concerns seem to oppose the promotion of women's health? First, we have learned to pay attention. That we had to remind ourselves to keep thinking about sex/gender during our observations in hospitals and at the transport company is evidence of how slippery the dragon really is.

Second, we need to become aware, in detail, of how exactly, in this workplace right here, equality concerns oppose the struggles for better health. Are there problems with equipment? with training? with colleagues? with supervisors? with managers? What kinds of solutions can align the two goals along the same path?

Third, we have learned to look and listen, and then look and listen harder and longer. Some of our interventions have led to mobilizing women and some have not. Why? We should probably get into the habit of separately consulting small groups of women and men. We tried this once, asking a male ergonomist to listen to a group of male teachers talk about keeping order in class. We learned that they were scared students would falsely accuse them of sexual touching, a fear we women had never noticed. But we have never dared to form groups of only women, although we have often consulted existing women's committees. We should consult women (and men) more explicitly. When it's not dangerous for them, we should consult racialized groups explicitly as well.

Fourth, what about our local interventions? How can we contribute to a dynamic that makes women stronger and healthier? Is Nicole right to keep explicitly political language out of her interventions and concentrate on the physical work environment? Her hard work in pushing for multiple small changes that improve health has certainly prevented disease among women workers in traditionally female jobs. She has also done some interventions that ended up reinforcing worker solidarity by getting rid of management practices that were causing tension among workers. There are probably fewer women crying in the workplaces where Nicole has intervened than in the French print shop or on our hospital wards. On the other hand, when we keep quiet about gender issues, it means that each woman worker is left alone to deal with them.

I think we should take a leaf from Nicole's book and go into more detail with our suggested solutions. It is not enough to say that the employer should work to eliminate discrimination against women and ethnic minorities. Uh-huh, says everyone, and goes on doing just what they were doing before. We need to find and try out concrete solutions like the anti-sexism training developed in France.[28]

Fifth, whatever we do, we need to develop and nourish solidarity among women, because that is what makes the other solutions possible.

Bottom line: I think we need to work globally toward a more feminist society. In the next chapter, I will describe how ergonomics intervention works with a feminist employer.

8.

FEMINIST ERGONOMIC INTERVENTION WITH A FEMINIST EMPLOYER

My friend Ana Maria Seifert was asked to teach hotel cleaning staff how to lift weights like mattresses more safely, but she ended up analyzing everything from work schedules to inter-ethnic relations.[1] Every study arises from a request from the workplace, but the study doesn't necessarily respond exactly to the initial request. Ergonomists try to figure out the basis for the initial request by interviewing critical actors, collecting information and records from the work site, and by preliminary observations of work. This process always leads to broadening or even transforming the potential area of concern. Best result: the ergonomists, workers, and employer representatives agree on the final questions. Ana Maria ended up enlarging the intervention, focusing not only on the weight of the mattresses the staff had to lift but also the resistance of the heavy carts they had to push along thick carpets, and even on the numbers of little bottles of shampoo and lotion they had to fill.

Usually we work with unions, but our 2003–2004 study of women's shelters came from a group of forty-three shelters that wanted to reduce "stress" and intergenerational tensions among counsellors. The workers were telling the association that they were

desperate, they wanted to quit. Some blamed their boards of directors, some their managers, some their older or younger colleagues,
some the provincial government for being stingy with funds.

The older counsellors (including those running the association) had founded the shelters at a time when conjugal violence
was not an accepted public concern. They came from all kinds of
backgrounds and had no formal training; many had been victims of
violence themselves. They had volunteered without pay, setting up
the shelters and running them with little or no financial or social
support. Some had been physically attacked or had seen colleagues
attacked or even killed in the course of their work. A counsellor
had been murdered by a resident's partner a few months before we
started our study, and the counsellors were still shaking in reaction.

Counsellors had never received much pay or social recognition.
Their pleasure in their work came entirely from their feeling that
they were helping other women and from the bonds they formed
with their clients and each other. They had pretty much invented
their counselling practices from scratch, developing and testing
methods of feminist intervention and original educational materials, with the support of their association. They complained that, for
the younger generation, counselling seemed to be just a job that
you trained for in a social work school. The younger women felt
stifled, forbidden to innovate or even to use the techniques they had
learned during their university training.

We gave 242 counsellors a standardized questionnaire used by
the province to measure Quebeckers' health. Yes, they were certainly
stressed, no doubt about it. Well over twice as many of them had
high levels of psychological distress compared to other employed
Quebec women their age.[2] An interesting paradox emerged at this
early stage of the study. When we looked at how the shelters were
managed, we could divide them into three groups: collectives run
democratically by all workers, shelters managed in a traditional

hierarchical way, and those where a hired "coordinator" organized the work in consultation with the employees. We were surprised to find the most distress among those in the collectives, even though their counsellors had more control over their working conditions.

But we needed to know more. What did the counsellors mean by "stress"? Where was it coming from? What stressors were they talking about?

We teamed up with Nancy Guberman, a professor of social work, to study the counsellors' assigned tasks. They had to help each woman to deal with her violent ex, of course, but they also had to make sure she and her children were fed, housed, and kept safe through court proceedings. Feeding involved meal preparation, grocery shopping, and cleaning up. Housing involved plumbing, repairs, and making sure children didn't make too much noise or fight with each other. Life is not simple, so some of the women had drug and alcohol issues that had to be dealt with as well.

Our preliminary observations vastly enlarged the list of job demands and required skills. Counsellors spent ever-increasing amounts of time preparing grant applications and asking for donations. They kept detailed records of interactions with residents and communicated them to other counsellors, but they had to keep the records safe from police or government officials who might use them against the residents. They had to collaborate with other government agencies, but they did not always get help from those agencies in return. In fact, they said the agencies showed no respect for the specific competence they had developed over years of dealing with partner violence.

Since most residents arrived in a state of crisis, counsellors faced new demands 24/7. Scheduling was typically established according to seniority, meaning that younger women, many of whom had young families, worked a lot of weekends and some nights. They mediated conflicts among the women and their children, all in crisis mode. In shelters with collective governance, counsellors talked with each other very often about how to handle problems with housekeeping, the board of directors, the law, the neighbours, and each other. With all these tasks, we wondered whether their working conditions allowed them to do what they saw as their primary job and their main motivation—counselling the residents.

During one of my first exploratory visits to a collectively run shelter, I observed an interaction between counsellors of different ages. Marie-Jeanne, the younger one, had gone out to buy supplies for a Christmas party and she had struck gold—she proudly told the older one, Barbara, about a decoration she had unearthed. Not only was it going to be fun for the children staying at the shelter, but she had gotten a bargain. Barbara used this opportunity to explain to Marie-Jeanne the importance of procedures and collective decision-making. Barbara was inflexible and took a stern tone. Marie-Jeanne's bargain was too expensive and she shouldn't have taken it upon herself to buy it without presenting her projected purchase at a meeting. Marie-Jeanne struggled with tears during the encounter, which ended with her leaving to take the decoration back to the store. I could see the intergenerational conflict being played out in front of me, and I got a feeling for why collectively run shelters could be stressful.

We ended up agreeing to work with the shelters on various sources of stress, including not only intergenerational issues but communication in general and time pressure.

Observing the work and asking questions

Observation is the key tool of ergonomists, and it is here that ergonomic studies distinguish themselves from those based on interviews. In fact, classic texts in francophone ergonomics employ the expressions "real work" (*travail réel*) as observed, to be contrasted with "assigned tasks" (*travail préscrit*).[3] The observations are oriented to produce a "true" and complete picture of the "real" work process, its determinants, requirements, and constraints.[4] The interviews we do complement and explain the observations.

The first observations help us figure out the work process. Usually this stage involves fifty to a hundred hours or so. We observe a variety of people, job titles, situations, and shifts. During this stage, we saw that sometimes a counsellor worked in physically constrained postures that seemed unhealthy and, at first, unnecessary. But the counsellor told us she had to position herself so that she could always see out of the front window of the shelter, because a dangerous ex-partner might show up. She showed us all the precautions she took to avoid being seen from the street, while seeing everything around her. We were introduced to all the complicated procedures surrounding the use of telephones and doors. What if a resident called her aggressor and, in a moment of tender reconciliation, revealed the location of the shelter? Or what if she opened the door to a violent not-so-ex-partner, putting everyone at risk? Observing made us aware of how much the possibility of violence conditioned counsellors' tiniest gestures.

We also learned about the practical implications of feminist principles. For example, all interactions with residents are considered to be potentially empowering, part of the healing process. Therefore there is no particular priority given to formal interviews with residents, as opposed to cooking a meal with them. Both are opportunities for support and empowerment. Although counsellors tried hard to spend formal time with residents, those interviews could be interrupted, and very often were.

We also learned about the sociopolitical context. We heard about a chronic lack of funds, leading to understaffing, low pay, and consequent rapid staff turnover. Some counsellors said they had trouble defending their work to skeptical friends and family. Those in a semi-rural setting felt exposed, since they were visible to their community and sometimes targeted as man-haters. Many said they never told people they met exactly what they did for a living.

We saw direct consequences of understaffing. Two counsellors scheduled a meeting to deal with a problem among residents. It was timed so that a volunteer could take care of the residents' children during the meeting. But one counsellor was on the telephone when the babysitter arrived and the other counsellor had to start the meeting alone. Then the other telephone rang and the second counsellor had to leave the meeting to answer it because any call could be a cry for help from a woman facing imminent violence.

When we asked why someone wasn't specifically hired to answer the phone, we heard different answers. Some had to do with funding, others were based on feminist principles (having only one "class" of workers rather than a hierarchy), and others on the needs of clients (having a first contact with people able to understand the caller's situation and act quickly).

Choice of situations to analyze in detail

Spending long periods of time with the workers is the part of ergonomics that I like the best. I am not very good at observing with my eyes, having a pathologically deficient visual memory (moderate prosopagnosia with complications), so I need students to help. But being with workers right where they do their jobs kicks and twists my brain into a new perspective. I can get a feel for how the shelters work, what the clientele is like, how life looks when you have to think about violence all the time. Questionnaires and interviews with the counsellors don't give me an understanding of the work as fast as walking into the shelter and seeing women covered with bruises, or watching a counsellor pacify some stressed-out women or children who are fighting. (Driving back from a shelter, I heard one ergonomics student say to another, after a long silence: "I was certainly right to break up with Bob when I did.")

After interviewing twenty-eight workers and observing in the shelters for fifty hours, we concentrated on two major areas. My colleague Céline Chatigny, with expertise in ergonomics and education, became responsible for an analysis of what skills were required of counsellors and how these were transmitted between generations; since schedules were another intergenerational issue, Céline took that on too. I was responsible for the study of communication, time use, and time constraints. Students Jessica Riel, Marie-Christine Thibault, and Eve Laperrière helped with the next observations and analysis.

Time use

No matter what generation they belonged to, all the counsellors wanted to spend their time counselling—that is, in direct interventions with the residents, preferably one-on-one. This was why they had chosen the job, what they liked about it, and what they felt best about doing.

> "It's when I do structured interventions that I really have the impression that I'm doing my job. Sometimes it can take several meetings before the woman can find her own way and when that happens it's gratifying for me, I feel useful." (day shift counsellor)

But our observations showed that they in fact spent less than half their time in one-on-one interactions with residents, and most of those were brief exchanges of information (Figure 8.1). They spent a lot of time, which we clocked at 14 percent, documenting what was going on with residents, in journals and written messages to other counsellors, and another 14 percent doing housekeeping and administration tasks like calling the plumber, making and serving meals, and paying bills. Depending on how many counsellors were present at the same time, they could spend another 13 percent of their time communicating among themselves.[5]

Another phenomenon we noted was the surprising number of interruptions. The median uninterrupted time for any task, from

Figure 8.1 Time use in women's shelters

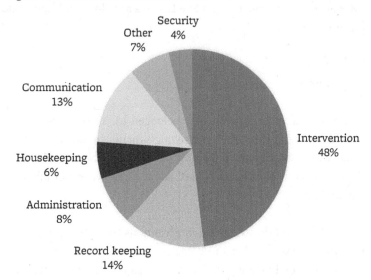

Source: Translated from Jessica Riel and Karen Messing, *Analyse ergonomique du travail des intervenantes en maison d'hébergement et de transition pour femmes victimes de violence conjugale : l'utilisation du temps,* report submitted to the Regroupement des maisons d'hébergement pour les femmes victimes de violence conjugale, April 28, 2005.

Aim	Activity	Average duration (minutes)	Median duration (minutes)
Security	Surveillance, answering door	2.2	2
Counselling (average duration 3.6 minutes)	Formal one-on-one discussions with residents	10.9	2
	Informal discussions with residents	3.8	2
	Telephone interactions	3.1	2
	Transmitting information	2.7	2
Record keeping	Notes, reports, records for the team	2.8	2
	Individual dossiers	2.5	2
	Phone call reports	2.7	2
	Developing personalized plans	2.9	2
	Personal notes	1.8	1
	Other (photocopies, faxes)	3.1	2
Administration	Management, finance	2.9	2
Housekeeping	Cooking, arranging repairs, cleaning	3.0	2
Communication	Communication among counsellors	4.0	2
Rest breaks	Breaks	4.3	2

Table 8.1 Duration before interruption of activities observed during 102 hours in three shelters with different managerial and regional characteristics

Source: Translated and condensed from Riel and Messing, *Analyse ergonomique du travail des intervenantes en maison d'hébergement et de transition*.

exchanges with residents to checking the door for security to dealing with phone calls, was two minutes (Table 8.1). Even the structured, individualized sessions sitting down with residents to discuss their situation only lasted an average of eleven minutes, and most were interrupted before two minutes had passed.[6]

Counsellors were interrupted by the phone, the door, the children, the women, and each other. During one formal counselling session between a counsellor and a resident, there were two interruptions by other residents and ten by fellow counsellors. We found that the work was quite different when counsellors were alone compared to times when another counsellor was present, so we observed both situations extensively and compiled numbers describing time use and interruptions in the two contexts. We realized that their fast work speed left the counsellors little or no time for relaxation or reflection. None of the shelters we visited had specified break times, and only the counsellors who smoked took regular breaks, most often sitting with residents who smoked. Although smoking time often involved forms of counselling, they still gave a change of pace—"I almost regret having stopped smoking," said one counsellor.[7]

Moving toward change

Counting minutes can lead to pressure for change. When we showed that direct counselling of residents was less than half of work time, counsellors said they wanted to increase this proportion. When we counted break time and found it to be way less than the legal requirement, counsellors agreed that they needed breaks. When we counted interruptions, we made the shelters aware of the problem.

Demonstrations can pinpoint aspects of the work that can potentially be changed. The problem elements are usually there for a reason. People weren't interrupting gratuitously. We found that there were fewer interruptions when there were more counsellors present to share the work, and we eventually recommended that counsellors work in pairs.

We could attribute interruptions to staffing policy (workers alone in the evenings compared with workers always or sometimes in groups), to feminist principles (all shelter workers are equal so all should answer the phone, cook meals, deal with the plumber . . .), to the threat of violence (constant awareness of surroundings, checking doors and windows). The discussions of our findings led to an ever-deepening understanding of the work activity, and to a lengthening list of determinants, whether in the workplace itself or in the surrounding context (e.g., inadequate financing, unfriendly neighbourhood).

At the same time, my colleague Céline was working with a residence that had an acute conflict about weekend work—older workers took advantage of their seniority to grab the weekday shifts, but many younger workers really needed to spend weekend and evening time with their young children. Solutions should ideally enlarge the workers' "operational leeway," their ability to control all aspects of the work. Here the shelters' commitment to feminist management came in handy. Principles of equality and social justice helped Céline broker a compromise that gave counsellors better control over their schedules. She also worked out some ways the younger counsellors could profit more from their elders' experience.[8]

What happens to recommendations

The association liked our report. They had us present it in small workshops at their annual meeting and they hired a journalist to write a version for public consumption. They used it both to train counsellors and to lobby the government for more money.

I recently ran into a young woman who was working at one of the shelters we studied—she had been given our twelve-year-old report to read when she started work. The association told us in fact that many of the current shelter workers had read it. When they met us, they even recognized the name of our research centre. As feminists, we were proud of having helped the shelters.

The association called us back in 2019, so we were able to see what had happened to our recommendations. During the intervening fourteen years, they had introduced changes based on the report, including fairer work schedules and better communications. The shelters gradually shifted away from the model of pure collectives and hired coordinators, while creating training modules on feminist management.

Unlike the situation with the hospital cleaners (chapter 3), our recommendations had not been forgotten. The shelters had been surprised at our statistics on interruptions, so they had followed our advice and promoted a policy of having at least two workers present at all times, one to be responsible for direct interactions with residents and the other for answering the phone and door as well as managerial and housekeeping tasks. The shelters had used our report to negotiate with the government for the money to pay the extra staff.

One of our recommendations had seemed to be really easy to adopt, but it turned out not to be. We had recommended that the time spent writing information in multiple documents be reduced by better computer-based document sharing, given that all the shelters had computers. But in some shelters, workers were unfamiliar with the use of the relevant software and some said they were (in 2005) reluctant to use computers; we therefore recommended to them that work shifts overlap for a period sufficient for the oral exchange of information. When we returned to the shelters in 2019, we were surprised to learn they were still complaining about all the notes they had to read and write, but still not sharing information by computer. Older and wiser, we realized that we hadn't fully understood the function of those information exchanges. Just as people who have witnessed a horrible accident or who have been attacked may tell their stories many times over to whoever will listen, many counsellors were using writing about their experiences to reduce their stress. They would tell the colleagues about how their days had gone orally, through daily reports, Post-its, and memos. One shelter manager told us that she was almost always glad to listen, but she was tired of plowing through pages of handwritten notes. Our task now is to figure out how counsellors can get the relief and comfort of sharing their stories without forcing others to read and reread the same information. And, more broadly, how to support the counsellors in their challenging jobs.

What made the intervention at least a partial success? I would say the first factor was the fact that the association really, really wanted its workers to be well and happy. It was joined in this by most of the boards of directors of the individual shelters. For once, the employer was on our side. Feminist solidarity was a job requirement for managers and workers, at the core of their "business model." Also, the managers were by and large self-selected to put the well-being of other women on a par with their own. Although some of the managers were better listeners than others, almost all whom we met struggled actively toward an ideal of feminist management. Finally, the counsellors were also very interested in notions of fairness and social justice and almost all applied these ideas to their own behaviour as employees.

But I have to emphasize the employer attitude, since it contrasts sharply with many of our other experiences with employers. The communications technicians' employer seemed entirely uninterested by the plight of the few women they hired, and certainly unwilling to spend money on adapting their jobs. The hospitals that employed the cleaners and health care aides didn't want to hear about the injustices we observed. The transportation company and the retail stores couldn't have cared less about work-family balancing. They were not being evaluated on that basis, and no one told them it was important—stockholders, scattered across many other cities, would vote management in or out based on phenomena with much clearer links to profits. Other researchers have tried to work with retail managers to make schedules more family-friendly, without much success.[9]

Those employers with the worst conditions do not necessarily want change, and the government agencies that oversee them are not necessarily helping. I recently gave a talk on workers' "invisible suffering" at a public health authority. After the talk, I was cornered by a group of public health service ergonomists. Their job was to observe work in businesses all over the province and to administer the public health programs—identifying occupational health problems and proposing solutions. They wanted to share their experiences with me, so we sat down in a small room in the basement. One after another, the ergonomists told me stories about finding terrible risks in workplaces but being unable to interest the employers in making changes. They were feeling sad, impotent, and guilty. I asked whether they could call in labour inspectors to order changes, but they said it depended on the inspector. Some would, but most wouldn't risk confrontation with the employer unless there was an immediate, dramatic threat to life and limb (more common in the men's jobs they had observed). And there weren't nearly enough inspectors anyway. (The occupational health authority's lack of enforcement was recently confirmed by an auditor general's report.[10]) So there was no incentive for the employers to improve the work environment. I had no suggestions for the ergonomists except to encourage them to do whatever they could. They told me to give more talks, so we cheered each other up a bit.

Thus, the shelters were not typical employers; they were actively engaged in promoting health among their employees, and their association was explicitly mandated to do so. We could talk about gender with them, since they were front-line feminists. There were no taboos on talking about problems; we profited from a free flow of information and ideas among the association, the workers, and ourselves. All possibilities were on the table, although many solutions we suggested turned out to be impracticable. There was a political process in place so that the shelters could themselves decide to implement solutions. There was also, most importantly, feminist solidarity among the shelter workers and their coordinators, fostered and nourished by the association. This was particularly important when Céline was working with the counsellors to make the weekend schedules fairer. Fairness and solidarity were in the DNA of the association and of the shelters.

I don't know whether the benign nature of the shelter association and the boards of directors, considered as employers, came from their feminism, the small size of each shelter, or the fact that the employer was a non-profit social enterprise. We did study another non-profit community-based living arrangement, and found more variability in the way their managers treated employees. Some were nice and some were nasty. Some had fair ways of setting up the work schedule and some were dog-eat-dog.

So feminist solidarity might be a model for management. Our own research centre, CINBIOSE, was set up by women with feminist principles and it has been led by feminists for over thirty-five years. The next chapter will try to show how feminist solidarity has helped us make changes in science and in our workplace, intended to help working women. Please forgive me for bragging; I am pretty proud of CINBIOSE.

9.
SOLIDARITY

n chapters 1 and 2, I gave some examples of how ferociously men can stick together when they feel women are attacking them. It would make sense that women being attacked would also want to support each other. But our experiences tell us there are powerful forces opposed to our getting together. I learned first-hand about the strength of those forces. When I went to work in my biology department in 1976, I became the second woman in a department of seventeen. My two (male) research collaborators lost no time in urging me to stay away from Donna Mergler, the only other woman, "for my own good." They said she wasn't well regarded; she was inconsiderate, not nice. Other colleagues echoed the warnings in similarly vague terms from time to time. Although I respected Donna as a brilliant researcher and an astute political analyst, I listened attentively to the guys and stayed away.

Over time, common interests began to bring Donna and me together. In 1977, the department that trained sex therapists (Département de sexologie) asked us and five other women professors to come to a meeting. They wanted us to participate in a program they were designing, because we had taught an interdisciplinary course in women's studies three years before.[1] They had already prepared the program and agreed on all the course content, but needed professors to teach the material. Since the sexology department, unbelievably, had no women professors, we could understand their need for help, but we rebelled at being called in as auxiliaries to a program the boys had fixed up without us. The late, brave sociologist Nicole Laurin led the resistance: "As a woman I am insulted!"[2] she exclaimed in her thrilling contralto voice, and we all walked out and started planning our own program, including courses on sociology, history, economics, and biology.

Donna and I went back to our department with a proposal for a course on women and biology. The department didn't make it easy; several of our colleagues were opposed to taking resources away from "disciplinary courses" like genetics and cell biology. But we united our forces and won, with support from students. And the course attracted students from outside the department, so our colleagues had to keep it.

Donna and I started spending more time together and each realized that the other was not as disagreeable as our colleagues had told us. Donna, who had not previously identified as a feminist but who has a well-developed sense of social justice, started giving me meaningful looks at key points during department meetings. When one of our colleagues proposed hiring "the little woman from Marseille with the musical voice" to teach a course, Donna was so far emboldened as to propose in jest that he be censured for sexism. But our colleagues had noticed our growing complicity and were not pleased. Donna's joke turned out to be the straw that broke the camel's back. Our colleagues started screaming and yelling at us. When they all stood up (Donna is five feet tall when stretched and I am not much bigger) we got scared. Luckily, Donna's office was just opposite the meeting room, so she and I raced out and found refuge there. But as we were pushing our door closed, the department chair and his buddies pushed against us to stop it. We felt the force of all those pushing on the door in our own bodies. We got the physical door closed, but our place in the department had changed forever.

We couldn't ignore the rage we had ignited and we had to figure out how to react. Donna and I became aware that, even before we had started working together, we had been perceived as the Gang of Two and there was no use pretending otherwise. We had to stick together, so we started having fun. I changed my research subject from fungal genetics to occupational health to work with her. By 1981, we had co-founded a research team that became officially associated with the government-run Institut de recherche Robert-Sauvé en santé et en sécurité du travail (Robert Sauvé Institute for Research in Occupational Health and Safety, or IRSST).[3] The IRSST generously supported us to do research on early indicators of biological damage incurred in the workplace, although it energetically resisted anything that sounded like research specifically on women workers.[4]

When IRSST abandoned its team grant program, Donna and I founded the CINBIOSE research centre in occupational and environmental health, which, under Donna's direction, became a World Health Organization–associated centre. Headed more recently by Cathy Vaillancourt, a cell biologist working on environmental damage to fetuses, CINBIOSE has thirty-seven member researchers, thirty-two of whom are women.

Solidarity and persistence have enabled CINBIOSE to help change government policy. The close association of ergonomics, biomedical, and law professors in solidarity with feminist labour, community, and environmental groups has been critical to translating research results into policy and practice around sexual harassment, violence, the work-family interface, protection of pregnant women and fetuses, the health of First Nations, environmental protection, and workers' compensation practices, for example. And researchers from CINBIOSE co-founded and directed UQAM's Institute for Health and Society, training young people to think about biology, psychology, and social forces at the same time.

Meanwhile, the group we started in reaction to the sexology proposal went (led by our colleagues in other faculties) from teaching a few courses on women to developing a multidisciplinary course program, a graduate studies program, a sustained collaboration with a consortium of women's groups (Relais-femmes),[5] and eventually an enormous institute for feminist research and teaching (Institut de recherches et d'études féministes).[6]

And what about the sexology department? I was elected to our union negotiating committee in 1979. Over the objections of some colleagues, we managed to put a clause in our collective agreement to provide for preferential hiring of women in departments with less than 40 percent women, along with actions to make it happen.[7] Our union women's committee then visited all the male-dominated departments that opened new professor positions, including sexology, to explain the clause and the action they needed to take. The departments didn't like it, but some of them let us talk to them, and some of them even listened. Today, after pressure from us and from other university feminists, women are 68 percent of sexology department professors. Our own biology department was not as successful, but it did develop from 12 percent when I was hired to its current 30 percent women.

Solidarity also helped us in our drive to make the IRSST understand the importance of gender in occupational health. During its first fifteen years, IRSST, governed jointly by unions and employer organizations, spent its research money primarily on jobs with very few women. This was the typical situation in occupational health at that time.[8] When we proposed a project on the health and safety of women blue-collar workers, with the support of their union, the union confederations supported us but had trouble dealing with the ferocious opposition from employers. The IRSST administrators who had helped us present the project found themselves caught in the middle. Again, I faced unexpected rage from both the embarrassed administrators and the unions. One male union negotiator cornered me alone with a litany about how I had injured the whole union movement by developing the project (with one of his unions)—an interaction that left me in tears. An official at IRSST publicly called me "stubborn as a mule" for persisting with my application and badmouthed me whenever he got the chance. I would probably have abandoned the whole project had it not been for the warm, sympathetic counselling and support of feminists in the unions. I will never forget my telephone exchange with Carole Gingras, the head of the Quebec Federation of Labour women's service, long after working hours. The position of her service in the union was not the most secure, but she supported me, and the other union feminists also wasted no time in patching things up between me and their hierarchies.

This whole episode left the IRSST shaking, even more afraid to support any research on gender and occupational health. When one of my PhD students phoned them to ask about access to scholarships for studying occupational health among immigrants, the program officer replied that no aid was available. "It's like research on women's occupational health," she snapped. "We don't support research on groups." In a letter confirming IRSST's refusal to examine the scholarship application, she said that "in [the Institute's] research priorities there is no policy on specific populations," and suggested that the student focus instead on "accidents, noise and vibrations, protective equipment, tool safety, industrial methods, chemical and biological agents, and musculoskeletal disorders." Only the last of these exposures is found with any frequency in women's jobs, which may explain why women were fewer than 15 percent of those covered by Institute-supported projects at the time, although women were 45 percent of the workforce. Dangers in women's jobs like sexual harassment and assault, variable and unpredictable work schedules, and prolonged standing were not studied. So CINBIOSE researchers published data showing Quebec government agencies understudied,[9] underprotected,[10] and undercompensated[11] women workers. I heard that the IRSST board was furious and even threatened the editor of a journal personally for publishing one of our (peer-reviewed) papers.

The union women's committees continued to fight to get support for women's occupational health. An expert in feminist survival tactics manoeuvred the law and ergonomics researchers into a union press conference on women's occupational health. Using data from our first studies, her union denounced the low priority given to prevention in women's jobs. The *Montreal Gazette* gave the event front-page coverage,[12] forcing the health and safety authorities to answer for some of their orientations and practices. And so it went, with political forces pushing back and forth inside and outside the government health and safety apparatus.

As we and others started to produce data on women's work, our partnership started to influence researchers at IRSST itself, some of whom courageously began to analyze their health and safety data with a gender lens; eventually this became their standard practice.[13] And the published provincial data banks on work accidents and illnesses started to include information on the gender of workers, making researchers' lives easier. Seventeen years after our first press conference, IRSST endowed a university chair to study gender, work, and health[14] and shortly thereafter, the Institute held an all-day seminar on the subject. They even invited me to speak. In 2017 they published a report on immigrants' occupational health that included gender considerations.[15]

Over the years, we found solidarity hiding away in various corners. In Ottawa, we discovered the Women's Health Bureau[16] of

Health Canada that gave us some money and respectability. One sunny day in 1990, Freda Paltiel, director of the bureau, asked me out to lunch. She wanted to know what she could do to help stimulate interest in women's occupational health among researchers and activists. I didn't have any idea, but she thought up something. She got her opposite number in the labour ministry to commission and publish the first government report on women and occupational health.[17] Then Freda and her troop of dedicated women's health experts sponsored a series of conferences on women's occupational and environmental health in the 1990s and early 2000s, attended by all kinds of scientists and practitioners—people whom the astute Freda had identified as influential. Susan Kennedy and Mieke Koehoorn from British Columbia made us aware of gender issues in epidemiologic analysis; Helen McDuffie of Saskatchewan told us about chemical exposures of farming women; Angela Tate, an engineering student from Newfoundland, explained to us that all of biomechanics research was based on male cadavers; and Pat Armstrong and her students at York University kept us up to date on social changes in the workplace. The conferences led in 1995 to the publication of a book with twenty-three chapters written by authors across the country,[18] as well as a collection of papers in a scientific journal.[19] These publications were critical to encouraging Canadian research and practice on women's occupational health.

Freda had a habit of getting women together whenever she could find an excuse, and her office kept up the practice after she retired. The meetings were relaxed, full of warmth and mutual support. A most wonderful thing for women happened at one of these get-togethers in the late 1990s, when Canada was setting up its Institutes for Health Research. Just the fact of us all together in the same room was enough to create the spark that led, after many battles,[20] to the Institute for Gender and Health. IGH not only stimulates and supports gender-sensitive research, but its energetic directors have pushed to make peer review for all biomedical research include questions on the inclusion of women and women's issues.[21]

Meanwhile, unions elsewhere in the world were becoming interested in women's occupational health because of the growing number of women in unions and the shift in men's jobs from manufacturing to the service sector, where their jobs were more like women's. The European Trade Union Institute, led by Laurent Vogel, commissioned our *Integrating Gender in Ergonomic Analysis* in 1999,[22] and got it translated into six languages by European unions and women's groups. Laurent has been organizing a series of international conferences on women, work, and health, bringing together researchers, unions, and community groups and reinforcing feminist research in Latin America and Canada as well as Europe. The 1999 Women, Work and Health conference in Rio de Janeiro developed interest in women's jobs in Latin America, and researchers are now active in Venezuela, Brazil, Chile, and Mexico. All this activity pushed women at the World Health Organization of the United Nations to commission an official WHO pamphlet on women's health and safety at work.[23]

Parallel movements were growing elsewhere. In 1994, a group of cancer researchers at the US National Institutes of Health focused on chemical exposures and their consequences and held several conferences encouraging inclusion of women in research on occupational cancer.[24] In 1998, the Swedish government sponsored a program called Women's Health at Work that stimulated research in both the social and natural sciences. In 2006, the International Congress on Occupational Health established its Women, Work and Health Scientific Committee. In the same year, the International Ergonomics Association set up its Gender and Work Technical Committee, initiated by CINBIOSE ergonomists and the French ergonomist group Genre, Activité, Santé. The technical committee has sponsored at least one daylong symposium at each triannual conference ever since. The 2021 conference has scheduled three symposia.

So solidarity among dedicated women has pushed occupational health and safety research and practice toward helping working women, against solid resistance. But nothing in this account should be interpreted as saying solidarity is easy or that Donna and I and our colleagues have been selflessly loyal to each other at all times. I remember dragging Donna into my feminist psychologist's office for couple therapy during the 1980s. Although it hadn't saved my marriage, the therapy worked for Donna and me. And it was worth it.

If there is a main message from the women's movement, it is that women have to believe in and support one another. It has been working in our department, at our university, with our funders, and in our scientific community. Union women's groups in Quebec have joined with feminist community groups on a cause-by-cause basis that has enabled us to resist attacks on protection for pregnant women and free access to abortion, and make great strides toward parity in government[25] and major improvements in pay equity. In my own studies with the group of women's shelters that prides itself on "women helping women" (chapter 8), I have seen solidarity yield practical returns in organizational harmony.

So, from my own experience, I would think that ergonomic interventions to transform women's work should fight denial and foster solidarity, but this is easier said than done. We need to analyze each situation as it comes up, and decide with our partners how we can best serve women's interests in each context. Is the union open to a feminist approach? Is the union strong enough to get ergonomists into the workplace or do we need to negotiate with the employer? Is it the right time for an attempt to change employer policies (about equipment or work-family balancing, for example)?

Is our current government open to introducing new laws? We need to make our decisions based on how to protect women at each workplace, while advancing the status of working women overall.

Mapping the dragon

What has our research during the *l'Invisible qui fait mal* partnership taught us about the forces that hurt women's health at work? From the research on women in non-traditional jobs, we have learned that women's bodies are the "second bodies" at work. Equipment, work site design, and training need to be adapted.

From the research on women's traditional jobs, we have learned that women's jobs are the "second jobs." They are badly paid, their requirements are underestimated, and their workplace problems are not recognized.

From our research on the work-family interface, we have learned that women's family responsibilities are "second roles," underestimated and not respected. Women have to jump through hoops just to get to work and they are accused of disorganization if they occasionally fail.

And from our research on women's occupational health, we have learned that women's health is "second health," understudied and badly studied.

If, as the #MeToo movement tells us, women need to name the aggression we face and hold responsible those who attack us, science is part of that naming. Scientific investigations have played a big role in deciding what health problems are recognized, how organizations deal with them, and who is allowed to speak about them. So Donna and I and our colleagues at CINBIOSE have been thinking about how to conduct scientific research that will help women, in collaboration with the women concerned and with their active participations.

Not all scientists have much contact or feel much affinity with working women. We have met denial, ignorance, and obfuscation during our research on women's occupational health problems. The next chapters will show some of our thoughts on how to deal with the dragons in science.

PART IV.
CHANGING
OCCUPATIONAL
HEALTH SCIENCE

10.
SCIENCE AND THE
SECOND BODY

J
ust to show you that scientists can sometimes behave like a bunch of guys in a bar . . .

In 2014, I posted a question on a sort of Facebook-for-scientists called ResearchGate, where researchers exchange information about their work. My question read, "Has anyone examined the effect of breast size on the biomechanics of lifting in industry or health care? Seems like women with larger breasts would have to carry objects further from the body, with effects on lifting efficacy (as well as back pain). But I can't find anything about this." Answers quickly appeared, all from men (we know their gender through the photos associated with their profiles).

1st researcher: There are some papers on this topic and [athletic] running. I don't know that I've seen one on lifting.

2nd researcher: I do not find any reason that similar females would have to carry objects further from the body. This would overload the lumbar spine. No matter if the breast size is large or small, they should lift and carry objects close to the body (under the breast). [Note: this answer can be counted on to make experts in biomechanics explode with laughter. If you are a woman, try carrying a box of, say, books, under your breasts.]

3rd researcher: If carrying something at waist height against the abdomen with the elbows bent at 90 degrees, it would seem to me that abdominal girth rather than chest size is the concern as this will increase the distance the object is positioned from the spine. So your question may be about females, but may also indirectly be answered in males. If a man has significant body fat, we would expect him to have larger abdominal girth. . . . I don't know how this would relate to breast size, except to say if an obese man has significant body fat, as evidenced by larger breast fat, we may predict he will have increased risk of back pain, due to the longer distance a load must be carried in front of the spine, because he will also have increased abdominal girth. [Again, peals of laughter from the biomechanics corner, since obese men do not have at all the same shape as normal women with breasts, and people don't usually carry big boxes at waist height.]

4th researcher: [Another irrelevant comment about running as a sport.]

5th researcher: *I have not studied the problem but have a solution for the problem* [my italics—this from a scientist!]. In Indian villages, women carry heavy weights, up to 30 kgs, on their back (packed in a basket or sack or bag) or on their head . . .

6th researcher: [This answer just repeats my question in more technical language.] It could be hypothesized that women with larger breast size would change the centre of gravity (COG) and line of gravity (LOG) anteriorly compared to women's with normal breast size or male population. The changes in COG & LOG may increase loading in back and hamstring muscles which may lead to altered efficiency of lifting.

7th researcher [I'll call him Carlos]: Joking and begging pardon if obscene, in Spain we say *"tiran más dos tetas que dos carretas"* [two tits pull (attract) more than two carts] . . .

8th researcher: Carlos, this is a good proverb. I got the meaning by the Google translator. Regards.

At this point I intervened and told them to forget it. While I can't compare this experience to a sexual assault, it did feel like my question, and I, and women in general, were being disrespected. It hurt, because my question was serious and I wanted answers. And it reminded me that the natural sciences, my work environment, is still in some ways a boys' club.

The second occupational health

Researchers have often treated damage to women's bodies as the "second health," and occupational health is no exception. By 1994, researchers like Jeanne Stellman, Vilma Hunt, and Shelia Zahm[1] had shown that women and jobs usually done by women were dramatically underrepresented in occupational health and safety research. In 1998, I suggested that this lack of knowledge had serious consequences for prevention efforts.[2] Figure 10.1 shows the "vicious cycle" affecting women workers as it existed at the time: a lack of knowledge about women's experience in the workplace led to interpreting women's occupational health problems as consequences of their biological or psychological "nature."

Because of these attitudes, women, even more than men, were discouraged from reporting work-related illnesses and found it hard to access workplace health and safety promotion, prevention, and compensation programs. Our problems remained invisible, cost little to employers and the state, and thus did not generate the kind of interest that stimulates research and identification of problems, thereby completing the vicious cycle. At the beginning of the twenty-first century, Isabelle Niedhammer and her colleagues showed convincingly that women were still excluded from occupational health research and that data on women's problems were

Figure 10.1 The vicious cycle in women's occupational health, 1998

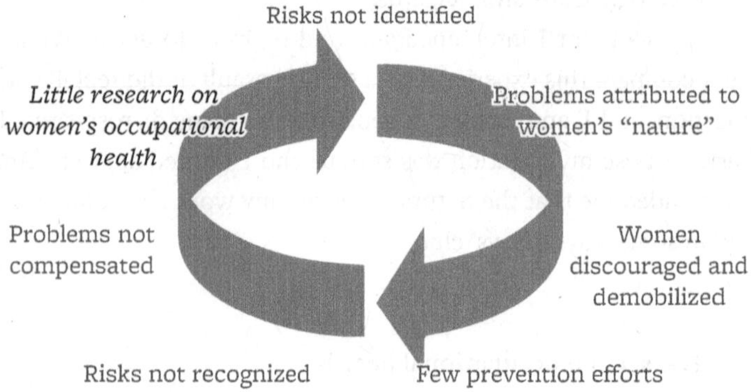

Risks not identified

Little research on women's occupational health

Problems attributed to women's "nature"

Problems not compensated

Women discouraged and demobilized

Risks not recognized

Few prevention efforts

Source: Adapted from Karen Messing, *One-Eyed Science: Occupational Health and Working Women* (Philadelphia: Temple University Press, 1998), 79.

seldom specifically analyzed.[3] In 2018, women were still catastrophically underrepresented in occupational cancer research.[4]

We also know very little about women's brains, and even less about how they respond to environmental influences. Women's brains (and those of female rats and mice) are much less often studied than their male counterparts,[5] and this exclusion from research may have consequences for prevention of pain and toxic effects among women. Donna Mergler found in 2011 that most workplace studies of the effects of workplace solvent exposure on the brain (the most common type of neurotoxic exposure) exclude women; more than three times as many studies include only men, compared to those including only women, although both sexes are exposed to solvents and can incur brain damage.[6] Donna looked again in 2019 and found only a slight improvement—the proportion of studies involving women went from 38 percent in 2002–2011 to 54 percent in 2012–18, and the proportion where the sex of participants was not reported went down from 26 percent to 15 percent. Most of the studies involving women still concentrated on environmental effects on fetuses, excluding the damage to the women workers themselves.[7] And there has been little research in the past decade on sex differences in reactions to other environmental neurotoxins.[8]

You may have noticed that no women responded initially to my question on ResearchGate. Maybe it was because they had nothing to say. But it is also true that many researchers, particularly women, don't like the idea of examining questions on male-female difference such as in types of strength, the effects of the work environment on menstrual periods, or the influence of sex hormones on reactions to workplace toxins. They have a very good reason—they are afraid that emphasizing sex differences will lead to stereotyping and eventually to discrimination against women. And, three months after I had left the (virtual) room, a young woman did respond, warning me that "this type of research might also result in women being shunned from the workforce," poetically adding "society . . . has not yet blossomed from the manure left behind from past sexual discrimination." She then wished me luck with my project.

Sex discrimination in science is not just a remnant from the past. We see it in peer review of women's grant requests,[9] our articles,[10] and our job applications.[11] And we see it in how scientists treat women's pain. So I think we also need to look that dragon in the face and measure its size, shape, and acceleration.

Sexism and work-related musculoskeletal disorders

In 2003, Katherine Lippel found that women's claims for compensation for musculoskeletal disorders were refused at the appeal level much more often than men's.[12] In Sweden, women are four times as likely as men to be denied compensation for musculoskeletal disorders.[13]

Some stories from injured workers remind me of what we are

hearing during the #MeToo movement. Descriptions of women's work-related pain are also received with skepticism, and women have trouble establishing their claims for compensation.[14] The experience of the claims process can even remind us of a violent sexual assault.

> "[The doctor] evaluated my ability to move my head, and he said to me, 'Can you turn further?' I said, 'No, I can't, it hurts me . . . I can't.' And then he took hold of me . . . he held me . . . he got behind me, he took hold of my shoulder, he took hold of my chin and he really forced the movement. . . . My knees gave out, and I started to cry, and it really hurt! But then he said, 'You're faking, it's not true!' And in his report he said that I complained about *any* movement." (woman worker describing a medical examination during her claim for workers' compensation, interviewed by Katherine Lippel and colleagues)[15]

The first problem, as with sexual assault, is a credibility gap. Sexual assault is rarely perpetrated in front of witnesses. Work-related pain, too, is not verifiable. It can only be reported by the person who feels it, not validated by any "objective" measurement. So if women report pain, their credibility is scrutinized. Are they exaggerating, dramatizing? Are they hypersensitive? When they describe their work environment, are they telling the truth? In interviews, claimants describe the same kind of mixture of hurt, loss of confidence, rage, and self-doubt.

> "We can't count on those around us for help. After all they don't know what you're actually experiencing. And living with chronic pain, nobody understands that either. They think that we make things up." (woman worker who

made a claim for workers' compensation, interviewed by Katherine Lippel and colleagues)[16]

To compound the difficulty, the fact that women are by and large excluded from jobs with obvious, dramatic dangers means that their work-related problems are harder to associate scientifically with their exposures at work. To make an association, epidemiologists need quantitative data; they need a large sample and, at the very least, unambiguous questionnaire items that describe the risk and the associated health problem. If a baggage handler at Transpeq has disabling backache, it is possible to show that it's because he was lifting heavy bags. We can count the bags and weigh them, or we can watch to see how often they lift.[17] If a cleaner has disabling backache because she spends long hours bending over to dust seats and clean toilets, the link is harder to make because there is no single weight to quantify, because it's too long and complicated to document all the different angles and strains on her back, and because their diverse relationships to back pain are harder to establish.

Another problem for women with work-related musculoskeletal (or other) disorders is a power imbalance. Women more often work in low-paying jobs. The low-paid woman reporting work-related pain is opposed by an employer who has many more resources and generally more advantages. Her union, even if it believes her, even if it thinks her problem is important, probably lacks resources to defend her, while her employer is supported by expensive white-collar professionals who are articulate and experienced in resisting claims.

Yet another problem is that women's bodies are the "second bodies" in the workplace, because women were a minority of paid workers when labour laws, work sites, labour policy, occupational health practices, occupational health science, family policy, and labour standards were being conceived. This late arrival has consequences: employers, doctors, and even colleagues don't know how to understand women's pain. Like many women exposed to repetitive movements, the French women at Florence Chappert's print shop (chapter 4) didn't develop their pain right away; it took several years for their manipulations of heavy books to create chronic inflammation. So the employer thought their complaints stemmed from their sex and age, and proposed hiring men as a solution. Indeed, a frequent defence against older women's claims for compensation for work-related pain is that the women are menopausal and therefore any health complaints are related to menopause, not work.

But, paradoxically, while sex-specific causes are invoked to avoid compensating women for their common work-related problems, women are not recognized or compensated for work-related conditions that are specific to us, such as aggravation of menopausal symptoms by poor environmental temperature control, fertility problems due to disturbance of menstrual cycles by shift work,[18] or intense perimenstrual pain due to poor work schedules, cold temperatures, or chemical exposures.[19] I have never seen a workplace prevention or compensation program that targeted female-specific problems, although some jurisdictions in other countries allow for unpaid leave during menstruation.[20] And breast size and lifting is not the only area that is underresearched because scientists are unwilling to deal with women's bodies. Where, for example, is the research on whether prolonged standing at work leads to urinary incontinence, given that standing may make our pelvic floor muscles work harder?[21]

When NASA scrapped an all-woman flight because they didn't have enough small spacesuits, it made headlines,[22] but the problem is much more general. Work stations, training techniques, and equipment are generally designed for the capacities, dimensions, and strengths of men's bodies, so a woman who has trouble after lifting weights can be told she is doing it all wrong rather than being given adequate equipment or being taught lifting techniques appropriate for her body shape, size, and centre of gravity. Work is organized to maximize the efforts of male bodies; it needs reorganization so as to profit from diversity.[23] Working in teams is good for men's backs as well as women's, but teamwork needs to be facilitated by such practices as assigning a group of patients to a stable team of hospital workers (rather than assigning each patient to a single worker who changes assignments every day) and by creating more regular work assignments.[24]

We also have to carry our struggles for recognition of women's pain back behind government policy, behind the workplace, to the obscure scientific and medical arenas where links are officially made between workplace conditions and women's pain and suffering. As we struggle to make a level playing field for women who have been sexually assaulted, we also need to adapt the ways science treats workplace damage to women's bodies.

This is not an easy task. For years, women have been excluded from study or badly studied.[25] Female-specific problems have aroused little interest. Little thought has been devoted to how to treat gender and sex differences in occupational health and safety research.

We need feminist researchers to think about sex/gender differences in work-related pain. In the next chapter, I will explain how we think about women's pain and, in the chapter after that, I will present some more general thoughts on how we occupational health researchers should treat gender in our analyses.

11.
UNDERSTANDING WOMEN'S PAIN

Stephanie Premji got her PhD with Katherine Lippel and me studying immigrant women and men working at a clothing factory in Montreal.[1] The union wanted to know whether and how immigrant status affected women's occupational health. At one of our first meetings with the workers, the local union representative was a sewing machine operator, originally from Haiti. She told us how she had sought compensation for her work-related shoulder problems: her symptoms, her difficulties on the job, and her struggles with the compensation board. Interspersed with her descriptions, she kept saying, "I'm not lying to you." As in, "it really hurt, I'm not lying to you" . . . "I had to stop working, I'm not lying to you" . . . "I had trouble making the beds at home, I'm not lying to you" . . . So I finally said I had no doubt she was telling the truth and asked why she would think we would doubt her. She answered that her neighbours, her family, even some of the other workers had trouble with the idea that working at a sewing machine could cause pain. It looked like such an easy job.

When Stephanie eventually compiled her results, she understood why the workers had pain.[2] They were paid on a piecework basis, meaning that they were paid a set amount for each piece of clothing they produced. So the immigrants, desperate for money to send to families in their home country, would work really fast, in cramped positions and making fast repetitive movements. They worked through their breaks and stayed on after their shifts. Then many of them, those who didn't absolutely have to go home to make supper and care for children, would go on to their evening language classes.[3] The endless days of overwork without rest turned into epicondylitis, shoulder tendinitis, and carpal tunnel syndrome. But their jobs didn't seem dangerous to their neighbours and family, or even to themselves.

When women reported sexual assault before the #MeToo movement, we encountered denial, mockery, and indifference. We complain too much or too late, we have contributed to our own misfortunes, we are making a big fuss about nothing, we haven't really suffered. Women reporting work-related pain run into similar obstacles: our pain is insignificant, it comes from our being too anxious, too fat, or too old, we are not working in the right posture, we got it from doing housework, we don't exercise enough, it's menopause, we complain about the tiniest little thing.

So how can feminist scientists study women's pain?

Work-related musculoskeletal pain—a common problem

Women workers suffer from work-related musculoskeletal disorders more than men, and this is especially true of women in manual jobs such as highly repetitive work in factories.[4] Seafood processing workers who dismembered and packed crabs during a short, intense season suffered terrible pain in their shoulders and arms that could only be relieved by heavy doses of medication.[5] Sewing machine operators, whose work site required them to hold trouser legs up high with one arm to feed the sewing machine, ended up with shoulder pain on that side.[6] But workers have been denied compensation for these injuries because the jobs aren't visibly dangerous. Post office workers picking up and sorting packages at the rate of one every three seconds have claimed workers' compensation for epicondylitis, but their claims were refused because the packages, at less than one kilogram each, were supposedly not heavy enough to cause pain.[7]

Just being confined to an uncomfortable posture can cause chronic pain over time. Receptionists, store clerks, and baristas who work long hours standing without access to seats develop pain in their backs, legs, and feet.[8] Office workers who bend their heads over keyboards can develop chronic shoulder and neck pain (and being sexually harassed may aggravate the neck tension and thus the pain).[9]

It is not only women who are exposed to repetitive tasks and uncomfortable postures that bring on chronic pain, but men's manual tasks usually involve exerting more force, with fewer repetitions per minute. Their risks look more impressive to the observer, and often lead to more obvious, more convincing damage. When women and men do similar tasks such as heavy lifting, both report a lot of accidents and injuries. For example, both women and men who lift, carry, and turn hospital patients have a high level of recognized work-related musculoskeletal disorders.[10]

Assessing pain

How can we answer the voices (sometimes in our own heads) that whisper or insinuate that women exaggerate, we fuss about nothing. Unfortunately there is not yet an "objective" way to assess pain.

A number of instruments are used to help people describe their pain, but they mainly come down to asking workers about pain frequency and intensity. Frequency can be assessed by "always /often / seldom / never" over a given period of time. Intensity can be reported on a scale (as from 0 to 10, where 10 is the most intense the person can imagine), or it can be assessed in relation to the ability to do common daily activities. Pain sensitivity can also be assessed, in pain-free individuals as well as those suffering from chronic pain. There are a number of ways to do this, like applying a measured amount of pressure to a defined body site and registering the pressure at which the individual first reports pain ("pain-pressure threshold").[11] But, in the end, all methods rely on the person reporting the pain.

All these factors together—the reliance on self-reports, the uncertainty surrounding the mechanisms that produce pain, the inability to relate the degree of pain to the tissue damage in a simple way—open the way to gendered, and often nasty, interpretations of the "reality" of people's experience of pain. Initially, when chronic pain was first associated with low-force repetitive work, some scientists called the phenomenon "hysteria," from the Greek word for uterus. They accused people complaining of pain from repetitive work of having a socially induced complaint.[12] Some specifically targeted women.[13]

What is musculoskeletal pain?

Musculoskeletal pain is associated with damage to muscles, nerves, joints, cartilage, and connective tissues like tendons and ligaments. It can be experienced as back pain, carpal tunnel syndrome (wrist pain), epicondylitis (elbow pain), osteoarthritis (joint pain), sciatica (lower back pain), or fibromyalgia (generalized pain felt at many sites), among other syndromes. Musculoskeletal pain is relatively common, reportedly the second most common disabling disease in the world (after mental disorders).[14]

Inflammation of tendons and muscles involves many genes, signalling systems, hormones, and environmental factors.[15] Scientists generally concur that chronic pain comes from interactions between the nervous system and the immune system, with a lot of steps intervening between what happens in the damaged body, to what (if anything) can be seen on an X-ray or other scanning device, to what is felt and reported by the worker.[16] Studies linking specific body damage to pain reports have not yet given us good information on what tissue changes exactly lead to musculoskeletal pain,[17] so there is a lot of room for invoking psychological factors and human subjectivity. Also, the transition between an initial, acute pain and chronic, disabling pain—critical in determining economic survival—is still being researched.[18]

Women's gender may also affect our access to care. Bottom line: we have to ask whether women's greater prevalence of chronic pain is partly due to a lack of medical knowledge about women's physiology, women's pain and its expression.[19] Deficiencies in diagnosis and treatment may force women to transition more often from acute to chronic pain. Women may have more chronic pain because their pain is inadequately treated and it doesn't respond to treatments conceived for men.

Maybe more research specifically on women's pain could also lead to better compensation of women's work-related injuries and illnesses.[20] Rejecting women's claims not only subjects the women to immediate economic hardship from lack of income, but also closes off access to help with rehabilitation.

Women's pain, men's pain—are they different?

There is already a consensus that women report more work-related pain than men. But there is a lot of controversy about how to interpret this phenomenon.[21] More specifically, what do scientists think may cause the male-female difference in pain frequency?[22] With musculoskeletal pain, evidence is starting to emerge that women and men (or at least female and male mice) may process pain differently.[23] The immune system mechanisms that have been identified for males may not be the ones that operate for females, but pain mechanisms have been very little studied in women.[24]

Studying gender/sex differences in pain can become very political, in part because of the same/difference debate (see chapter 5). There is a lot of palaver about whether women's and men's brains are *congenitally* different, and to what extent.[25] To me, this is not an important question, since everyone agrees that brains are plastic; that is, they change with experience. So any differences in experience will be reflected in the brain, and it would be surprising if adult women's brains and nervous systems did not show any differences in form and function from those of men, on average, whether or not the differences are inborn, hormonally determined, and/or influenced by gender roles.

Pain at work

Among Quebec workers, many more women than men report work-related pain that has "interfered with their usual activities always or most of the time during the preceding year."[26] The 2007–2008 EQCOTESST study (Enquête québécoise sur des conditions de travail, d'emploi, de santé et de sécurité du travail) of the Quebec population found that 25 percent of women workers, but only

16 percent of men, suffered from these work-related musculoskeletal disorders.[27] Seven years later, the Quebec Survey of Population Health raised those estimates to 31 percent versus 20 percent,[28] and the 50 percent excess of women was still there. Why was this? Are women working closer to their physical limit?[29] Is it because there are fewer prevention efforts in our jobs? Do we indeed complain more or earlier? Or are there other explanations?

The risks associated with traditionally female jobs tend to be diagnosed as illnesses rather than accidents. Repetitive manipulations and fine, precise movements slowly and undramatically lead to upper limb musculoskeletal disorders like carpal tunnel syndrome and epicondylitis. Prolonged static standing (think receptionists, grocery checkout clerks, baristas) generates pain from circulatory problems, backache, and swollen ankles and legs.

The ratio of about 1.5 women per man affected by work-related musculoskeletal disorders is seen in many studies, although the ratio varies somewhat by body site. Men have more knee pain, perhaps because they move around more often at work; women more neck pain, perhaps because they more often work long hours in static positions in front of a screen and/or because the dimensions of their office equipment are too big for them.[30]

Bad design is not the only problem. Recall also that women and men working for the same employers at the same jobs in cleaning and restaurants are exposed to different working postures. Even within the same classification or name of an exposure such as "repetitive work," "lifting weights," or "prolonged standing," men and women are exposed differently. Men who lift weights tend to lift heavier weights, and the heavy weights women do lift tend to be (wiggly, resistant, inconveniently shaped) people; women's repetitive work is also more so than that of men (i.e., more movements per minute); women who stand are less often able to move around than men who stand.[31]

We also learned from the EQCOTESST study that twice as many men as women reported occupational accidents serious enough that they had to lose time from work.[32] Are employers more at ease with exposing men to danger? Do men accept "danger pay" more often because of their economic responsibilities? Are men more careless? Do they take their accidents more seriously? Are they freer to take time off work when they are hurt, either because they are better paid or because they do not go home to an excess of domestic tasks?

Part of the answer is that traditionally male jobs in construction, forestry, and mining more often lead to visible, dramatic accidents such as falls, burns, and cuts.[33] Since men more often lift very heavy weights, they are exposed to a higher probability of acute back problems whose link to the workplace is more obvious. And men's social roles in male-dominated jobs like police officer, barman, and soldier can subject them to physical violence (although there is also increasing violence toward women in service-sector jobs like health care and sales). The link between a disability and a visible accidental event or a violent attack is easier to establish than with a long-term, low-level exposure. So it is easier to gain recognition and compensation for accidents than for illnesses. Unions are naturally inclined to concentrate on the life-threatening conditions in men's jobs.

But eye-catching conditions are not a good way to decide on occupational health research priorities. Scientific data are used to decide on prevention programs as well as decisions on compensation for work-related pain, and right now women are not getting their fair share of either prevention or compensation.[34] How can and should we study women's and men's work-related musculoskeletal problems in order to attain health and equality in the workplace?

12.
THE TECHNICAL
IS POLITICAL

When I went to France in 1990–91 to learn ergonomics, I had lots of time on my hands after my classes. So I went to visit my friend Marie-Josèphe Saurel-Cubizolles, who worked at Inserm, the French national medical research institute. I wanted to learn enough about epidemiology, the statistical study of population health, to understand articles about occupational health problems. I had come to understand that epidemiologists wield a lot of power in deciding where and how to prevent illness. Because they analyze large data banks using strict rules and procedures, they get to identify what factors cause illness. For example, they have a deciding influence on whether or not a worker exposed to a particular condition or chemical will be compensated for work-related cancer.

So I was particularly interested in how gender was treated during epidemiological studies of workers' health. At Inserm, they had a data bank from questionnaires about work and health in the poultry processing industry. Marie-Jo and her colleagues, who shared my interest in gender, kindly gave me an elementary understanding of epidemiological analysis, opened the doors of their data bank, and set me up with a computer. I am going to explain here how I realized that statistical analyses have political importance for transforming working conditions and how I found out that some analytical strategies have booby traps for women workers.

Why we want to separate women and men in our analyses

At that time, the standard way to analyze data on women and men was to line up all the possible exposures in a work environment (chemicals, temperature, movements, work schedules, and so on) and assess them, either by environmental assessments of some kind or by asking workers to fill out questionnaires. Then the scientists would evaluate the workers' health, again either by asking them questions or by medical procedures. The epidemiologists would then cross the data on exposures with the data on the health risk they were interested in to see whether any of the risks were associated statistically with the health problem. If the risk was associated with the health problem, they needed to think about possible ways the risk could cause the health problem. Eventually, when the scientists were sure that the risk caused the health problem, they would call for prevention by eliminating the risk.

But if the epidemiologists had reason to believe that an exposure-disease relationship might be spurious, influenced by (for example) the workers' gender, age, ethnicity, weight, or smoking behaviour, they would introduce a procedure called "adjustment." They would "adjust for gender" by making a mathematical correction that would render data on women and men more alike, so as to isolate and reveal the specific relationship between exposure and disease, minus whatever confusion might occur due to biological or other differences between women and men. For example, if they wanted to see whether working with dull knives was related to musculoskeletal problems, *and* if women in the poultry processing plants generally had more such problems than men, *and* if women were also more likely to be working with dull knives, the computer program would be told to correct the relationships between dull knives and musculoskeletal problems. That way, the strength of the specific relationship between dullness and health could be appreciated without the complications introduced by gender. The underlying idea here is that, somehow, being a woman or a man could cause the disease by some other mechanism than the dull knives, so we want to get rid of the proportion of the disease "caused" by gender and just look at the dull knives.

Both Marie-Jo and I wondered about this procedure. My ergonomics courses had made me observe workers carefully, and I had seen that two people could say they were exposed to the same questionnaire item (exposure to "prolonged standing," "cold temperatures," "dull knives") but their real exposures could be completely different. For Jeanne, "standing" was standing still in a cramped posture all day, while for Pierre, "standing" was walking around from time to time and sitting down for a couple of minutes whenever he got tired. For Anne, "cold temperatures" were sitting all day at an assembly line cutting up chickens at 4 degrees Celsius, while for Paul, "cold temperatures" were walking in and out of a freezer set at minus 20 degrees Celsius, several times a day. And Marie's "dull knife" was usually a lot duller than Luc's, because no one had told her how to sharpen it.

So Marie-Jo and I were afraid that "adjusting for gender" might really mean cancelling out all of women's and men's unmeasured differences in working conditions, thus destroying the whole point of the analysis. With the help of France Tissot, a statistician, we were able to demonstrate that, as Nicole Vézina and Donna Mergler had already told us,[1] women and men had very different working conditions. The women more often made very fast repetitive motions, had ill-adapted work stations, and experienced cold and drafts, while the men stood more often and were more often exposed to irritating gas and to extended and unpredictable work schedules.

We then demonstrated that both women and men were absent from work for musculoskeletal problems, but not for the same reasons (middle two columns of Table 12.1). In fact, neither of the risks for men appeared to be a risk for women, and vice versa. Women risked musculoskeletal problems if their work station was badly adjusted and if they had to exert an effort. Men risked those problems if they had a poor relationship with their supervisor or if they were exposed to humidity.

If we had used the procedure of "adjusting" for gender (as we did to produce the right-hand column of Table 12.1), several risks would have been underestimated for both genders and one (humidity, for men) would not have been identified. Yet men exposed to humidity were more than twice as likely (2.2 times) to be absent for a musculoskeletal problem.

What was striking about the study was that no one would have noticed the relationship with humidity for men had the gender-separated analysis not been done. The relationships between musculoskeletal problems and the other factors would also have been underestimated.[2] And no one would have noticed anything wrong, because there was no significant difference between these women and men in the incidence of musculoskeletal disorders.

Why are the relationships different? Why is humidity only important for men? It might be because of a sex difference in the reactions to humidity; it might be because humidity is a problem only for certain operations done by men, making objects slippery, for example. Or it might be that only one corner of the building is humid and that happens to be the area where men do a particularly dangerous set of operations. I don't know, and by the time we figured all this out, I was far from the French poultry processing plants where we could have explored these questions.

Table 12.1 Risks ("odds ratios") associated with at least one absence during the previous year for musculoskeletal problems, reported by women and men in French poultry processing plants			
Possible risk factor	Extra risk of absence associated with the factor, for women	Extra risk of absence associated with the factor, for men	Extra risk of absence associated with the factor, for both genders, adjusted for gender
Work station not adapted for worker's dimensions	2.8[a]	Could not be calculated because too few men were exposed to this factor	1.8
Effort exerted with arms	2.4	No significant relationship	2.0
Poor relations with supervisor or colleagues	No significant relationship	3.1	2.5
Uncomfortably humid at work station	No significant relationship	2.2	No significant relationship
Female gender	–	–	No significant relationship

a Means that women with ill-adapted work stations were 2.8 times more likely to be absent for musculoskeletal disorders than women whose work stations were adapted for their dimensions.

Source: Karen Messing, France Tissot, Marie-Josèphe Saurel-Cubizolles, et al., "Sex as a Variable Can Be a Surrogate for Some Working Conditions: Factors Associated with Sickness Absence," *Journal of Occupational & Environmental Medicine* 40,3 (1998), 250–60.

But we did gather together a group of recognized occupational health scientists to think about work-related musculoskeletal problems and gender, and we agreed that it was important to do analyses separately by gender. We published a paper together that was cited over two hundred times in the following years, a large number of citations for a paper on occupational health.[3] This probably means that more people are separating women and men in their epidemiologic analyses. Is this a good thing?

Mechanisms and standpoint

In order to answer that question, we need to think like scientists. To prevent disease, we have to understand as much as we can about the *mechanisms* underlying the production of the disease. So, in order to understand how to prevent the musculoskeletal disorders we found among men exposed to a humid environment, we need to look at other humid environments, look in the laboratory at how muscle tissue reacts to humidity, better characterize the humid environments in poultry slaughterhouses.

This emphasis on mechanism is particularly important in scientific studies of sex/gender differences in the workplace, where there can be a tendency to report such differences blandly, as they are found, feeding into gender stereotyping (see below). That is where scientific *standpoint* comes in. Health scientists have long debated the meaning, feasibility, and importance of scientific "objectivity." Positions range from critiques of the notion of objectivity itself[4] to descriptions of bias in the scientific treatment of certain groups[5] to generation of rules and practices meant to guarantee objective presentation of data.[6] In 2010, health researcher Joan Eakin suggested that "standpoint" may be a more useful and less polemical way to describe public health research practices.[7] The standpoint or point of view of the researcher can be critical for the choice of topic to study, phrasing of the research question, methods, interpretation of data, and communication of results.[8] And everyone has a standpoint, whether or not they describe themselves as "objective." For most CINBIOSE researchers, our standpoint is that we want to promote women's occupational health and gender equality in the workplace. From that standpoint, there are both advantages and disadvantages to separating data on women and men.

A downside of separating women and men in statistical analyses

After we published our articles on separating female and male workers in data analyses, we were happy to champion this cause. But after a few years, problems started to come up. The first was that some scientists started just reporting male-female differences without seeking to explain them. The researchers sometimes cited our papers to justify separating women and men uncritically in their analyses. This was particularly an issue with psychological effects of work, where there is a historical tendency to portray women's heads as especially weak and complicated. We didn't like to see bald-faced statements like "men in our study reported more problems with supervisors while women reported more anxiety." We were afraid that our statistical technique might encourage gender stereotyping.

We had wanted to further understanding of the health risks of women's jobs as well as men's, but separating women and men without thinking about the mechanisms at play is not a good idea.[9] We don't want to stimulate a lot of publications saying *without further investigation* that "women workers exposed to solvents are more subject to depression than men" or "women workers whose

foremen don't support them are more often psychologically dis-
tressed than men in a similar situation." Come on, authors, are you
sure that the men are really in a similar situation?

Mélanie Lefrançois, our authority on work-family interactions,
brings up the converse problem: When we separate women and
men and find no differences, we have to look further, too. We can't
be sure that the same work schedule or job title or state of fatigue
has the same meaning for a mother of four and a father of four.
In sum, we are all for exploring the mechanisms that underlie sex/
gender differences in occupational health, but we don't see the
use of making lists of differences. Such lists may even be harmful
because they carry a risk of stigmatizing women.

A second problem is even more complicated to solve. Gender
is not the only population descriptor that affects exposures at
work; for example, being an immigrant worker affects occupational
health,[10] as does being a member of a visible minority[11] or coming
from a less privileged economic class.[12] And women and men differ in their occupational exposures within each social category; in
Quebec, immigrant women face different challenges from immigrant men.[13] But examining occupational health risks separately for
categories like Indigenous men, Black immigrant women, or young
Hispanic women would, in most studies, make the sample sizes too
small for statistical analysis.

Luckily, I got to the 2008 Women, Work and Health conference
in Zacatecas, Mexico, and heard Annika Härenstam's keynote talk.[14]
Annika, a well-respected Swedish researcher, said she had decided
not to separate her studies by gender anymore. I was shocked, since
I knew Annika well and thought she cared about women workers.
But then her argument started making sense to me. She was saying that since women and men were not totally different but just
somewhat different, it was better to analyze working and living
conditions first and then see where the women and men fit into

different groups of conditions. She and her colleagues had done this with questionnaires filled out by Swedish municipal workers.[15] The people reported on all the risks in their jobs and on their personal situations.

First, Annika and her collaborators looked at the job characteristics. They found that some of the characteristics occurred together. So, by mathematical tricks, they divided the workers into groups according to their answers. People with physically strenuous jobs were in one cluster, and people who had to care for people were in another. She gave the groups evocative names like "physically strained" and "onerous human service job." Then Annika looked at each of the groups to see where the health problems were and where the women and the men were to be found (they didn't look for immigrants or racialized groups, but they could have). With no surprise, she found that the women were in the clusters where the conditions and health problems were worst.

Annika then examined each cluster to see exactly where the people worked. In this crafty way, without mentioning gender, she could name specific municipal services that needed to change. Her population being the heavily unionized Swedish public sector, the services listened and women's conditions were improved. Annika's message was that her statistical approach ("cluster analysis") made it possible to avoid gender stereotyping and hitting at people's sensitivities but still improve conditions for women. Her method has the advantage that any number of population descriptors can be projected on the clusters, with no limits on how few people fit the descriptors: we can ask where the trans women, the immigrant men, and the less-educated older people are. After this kind of exploratory study, we can then concentrate on the groups with problems and identify the specific risks we want to change, and we can also identify and attack the discrimination that puts certain groups in the worst conditions.

With France Tissot and Mélanie Lefrançois, we tried out Annika's approach with our data on work-family balancing among retail sales workers.[16] This was the study I mentioned in chapter 7, where we were kicked out of the workplace for being too interested in women with families. We wondered whether we would have had more political success with a cluster analysis. So we tried it out—we clustered the workers according to the constraints they experienced and found two clusters with a lot of constraints and two with relatively few constraints. We found that the older women with families were found in the cluster with a lot of work-family needs, and that they were the least happy with their jobs. But the cluster didn't only have women in it; men were 40 percent of the cluster. Thus, changes in the schedules would help a lot of women and a good number of men. Would the employer have listened if we had shown him the cluster analysis rather than the male-female analysis? Maybe, because he was more interested in the men.

There are an increasing number of innovative statistical techniques that may do a better job of both representing data and suggesting action, and we need to think more about them.

The political importance of technical decisions

The Institute of Gender and Health of the Canadian Institutes of Health Research (CIHR) has been trying to persuade medical researchers to include female research participants since it was born in 2000.[17] They started by simply asking researchers to state whether they included females in their samples. They advanced, a few years later, by asking researchers who did not include females to explain why not. Then they made it mandatory for many CIHR grantees to include a researcher knowledgeable about sex and gender on their teams. Nevertheless, the argument about whether and how to include women—and female rats and mice—is still going on, in Canada and elsewhere.

The people who work at CIHR told me about a problem they were having. Scientists were saying they didn't want to use gender-sensitive data analysis techniques because it would lessen the power of their statistics to find significant results. They said the ones who worked with animals didn't want to have to buy more animals for their experiments, and the ones who studied workers didn't want to restrict their studies to big workplaces. I made the rash statement that the scientists might be wrong, that thinking about gender might in fact *increase* statistical power. People got excited when I said this, so we had to undertake a project to explore whether, why, and how much this might be true.[18]

Statistical power to detect an effect is really important in occupational health studies, because dangerous workplaces are often small, but the danger may be high. If microelectronics workers seem to be getting dizzy and confused more than other people, I want to find out about it *right away* so I can push the employer, "Cutest Phones Ever" (CPE), to identify the guilty solvent and remove it from the workplace before the workers' brains are permanently injured. But before CPE is going to spend time and money on cleaning up, they want to be convinced that their workplace really causes cognitive damage. To convince them, I need to show that the people exposed to the chemical do worse on a validated test of cognition than people not exposed.

It will be a lot easier to demonstrate a risk at CPE, a giant factory employing a thousand workers, than at neighbouring "Funky Yellow Mobiles" (FYM), a startup with only ten workers. In Table 12.2, I show the results of a tenfold increase in the risk of brain damage in a large group versus a small group of workers. The result: we can statistically demonstrate the risk for the big company but not the

Table 12.2 Fictitious example of the inability to identify risks for small samples, even when the risk is the same as for big samples

Cognitive impairment	Work for CPE	Work for FYM	Same city but no chemicals at work	Work for CPE Women	Same city but no chemicals at work Women	Work for CPE Men	Same city but no chemicals at work Men
Damaged brain	100	1	10	50	5	50	5
Intact brain	900	9	990	450	495	450	495
Excess risk	10-fold	10-fold	Comparison group	10-fold	Comparison group	10-fold	Comparison group
Probability that the exposure is *not* associated with a damaged brain	Less than 0.0001, Fisher's Exact Test	0.1042, not significant, Fisher's Exact Test	This is the control group to which the others are compared	Less than 0.0001, Fisher's Exact Test	This is the control group to which the other is compared	Less than 0.0001, Fisher's Exact Test	This is the control group to which the other is compared

small one. Dividing the sample by sex doesn't change these results, if there are still a lot of women and a lot of men in the samples.

So analyzing big numbers is important, and scientists have objected to including women in their studies because they think it would mean either doubling the size of their sample (too expensive) or halving the number of men and therefore, in their eyes, diminishing the likelihood of finding any results. This argument is not always valid since our study of poultry workers (Table 12.1) showed that thinking about gender and dividing the sample by gender could in fact *raise* the likelihood of finding an association, when the mechanisms at play are different for women and men. But there has been prejudice against including women.[19] As one well-respected cancer researcher put it to me, "Women don't get occupational cancers, so it isn't cost-effective to have them in our samples." Well, Mr. Scientist, number one, women do so get occupational cancers. Researchers have shown that exposures to rotating night shift work[20] and various chemicals[21] have been associated with women's breast cancer, for example. And number two, just so you know, researchers have been studying occupational origins of male breast cancer, an exceedingly rare disease, since the 1990s.[22]

The result—CIHR is including sample size in a series of "Fact sheets" on how to treat sex and gender in health data analysis, and why paying attention to sex and gender can improve the likelihood of finding what causes disease.

Making decisions

The purpose of statistics is usually an aid to decision-making. In the phone company example, we decided that working at CPE was associated with brain impairment because a statistical test showed that there was less than one chance in ten thousand (0.0001) that the exposure was *not* associated with a damaged brain. With results that dramatic, the CPE union will want to get right on the problem. The workers will insist on better ventilation, want to put covers on the vats full of solvents, maybe even wear masks.

But suppose the results are less dramatic, as they very often are. How much risk can we tolerate before starting action? R.A. Fisher, an early statistician, arbitrarily set the limit at one chance in twenty. He suggested we consider that there was an association if we had less than one chance in twenty of being wrong. But if I worked at FYM (see Table 12.2), I would be unhappy about that probability of 0.1042, meaning that I had just over one chance in ten of being wrong in mobilizing for ventilation, vat covers, and masks. I would still want to mobilize everyone to help lower my exposure. So statistical tests are an aid to decision-making but not a substitute. I will definitely want to discuss the FYM situation with my co-workers, and maybe we will join the picket line at CPE.

Something tells me that my boss at FYM will have another point of view. Like the managers at the French printing facility in chapter 4, he may not think that the brains of a bunch of women workers are worth much. When my boss chats with his pals at CPE, they are going to want the study to be done over again (and again) before they are sure they want to spend money on cleaning up the environment. Even one chance in ten thousand may not be enough to convince them. In the context of workers' health, technical issues merge with economic and social choices.

A risky venture—measuring sex and gender

In the previous examples I treated sex/gender as a single, binary variable. But more and more people are considering both sex and gender as separate complex constructs. So some scientists are examining ways to measure sex and gender as continuous variables. The idea is that sex and gender are not dichotomous, that people have a range of hormones, body shapes, abilities, appearances, and psychological characteristics (for example) that can't be unequivocally associated with being *either* male *or* female, masculine *or* feminine. The next logical step for quantitative health scientists seems to be to measure sex and gender, to get a score for each person along a continuum from male to female or masculine to feminine so as to be able to assess the effect of sex or gender on health.[23]

In occupational health, some highly respected scientists have proposed a gender measure based on certain information available from the Canadian Labour Force Survey.[24] These authors are working from a standpoint I agree with: they want to improve the health of women and men in the workplace, and they want to understand the role played by gender in determining health. They gave participants a higher (more feminine) score if they reported absence from work or working shorter hours due to personal or family responsibilities; worked in an occupation with more women; worked fewer hours relative to their partner (presumed to be of the opposite sex/gender); or had a lower educational level relative to their partner. So being more like a woman meant taking family responsibilities seriously, working with other women, and having a husband whose career could be considered to be more important (although they didn't actually know they were dealing with only heterosexual couples).

Wait a minute—I have a problem with this approach, even aside from the stereotyping. Generally, the reason population health scientists want to associate risk factors quantitatively with health outcomes is to improve health. You find out asbestos exposure is associated with mesothelioma, a type of cancer? You try to keep people from being exposed to asbestos. The reason this works (and it does) is that there is a *mechanism* involved—the asbestos fibres are breathed in, they cause lung cells to die, and the cells release toxic proteins that transform lung cells into cancer cells.[25]

Knowing the mechanism is the basis for intelligent prevention. You find out that breast cancer is associated with night shifts? You think the mechanism has to do with too much exposure to light over too many hours? You explore whether dimming the lights or sending health care aides into dark places for breaks will help. But maybe the mechanism has (also?) to do with night work messing up biorhythms, leading to overeating and overweight. So then you would want to look at giving people lengthy meal breaks so they can have sit-down meals and having low-calorie snacks available at the nursing station.

How would this work with gender? Supposing we find that the higher (more feminine) people score on a gender measure, the more likely they are to die in the next five years. How would knowing this prevent their deaths? What is the public health message? Would we want to send them on courses to become more masculine? Or would we just have to break down the gender measure to figure out which component actually caused the health effects? Was it their family responsibilities? working in a segregated occupation? feeling oppressed? Aggregating people's labour force experience into a measure of gender seems to go in the other direction from figuring out mechanisms.

And of course I am not happy about promoting stereotypes concerning occupational health. I had a conversation not long ago with a scientist I usually admire a lot, so I won't name her here. She was working hard to develop a measure of gender that included a unit on the workplace. Two of her items asked about lifting weights and repetitive movements. Lifting weights was scored as masculine and repetitive movements was feminine. If you remember, in North America, lifting weights is now associated with male occupations only if the weights are not human beings, and repetitive movements are now associated with female occupations only if they are relatively fast movements. So she should have been careful about what she called "repetitive" or "weights," because movements at work can be complex.

But, beyond that, the exposures are associated with one or the other gender in a specific time and place. A new employer moves into the city and hires men to enter code into computers. What do you know, the men's scores for gender go up to resemble women's because they are doing more repetitive work. Really? We are getting a long way away from any mechanisms associating risks and health. And who wants to encourage reifying the association of repetitive movements with being feminine? It seems paradoxical to score exposures in binary categories in order to counter binary thinking about gender.

On the other hand, identifying people as one sex or gender rather than another (as opposed to trying to measure the exact degree of either gender) is important when identification with a specific sex, gender, or type of gender nonconformity is a source of oppression or power in the workplace. The work of Greta Bauer and her collaborators is important in producing reliable, non-exclusionary self-identifications that can be used in health surveys.[26] That said, Bauer is the first to point out that gender is less an individual characteristic than a social relationship, so we need to be careful how we think about classifying it.[27]

Ergonomic analysis and gender

Ergonomists analyze work and each job should be analyzed as part of an ecosystem composed of a work station, other work stations with which the worker interacts, the rest of the workplace, and the social, political, and physical environment surrounding the workplace. The work activity is a seamless integrator of all the elements of the ecosystem.

Gender, like age, minority status, and social class, pervades the entire ecosystem. Like the other qualifiers, gender is simultaneously an individual characteristic, a determinant of work activity, and a determinant of interactions with many other elements of the ecosystem. Paradoxically, although gender and sex are inseparable from and flow into work activity at many points, gender/sex discrimination is a binary process and usually acts specifically against women, just as racism specifically affects racialized populations.

Integrating gender, immigrant status, and so on, into ergonomic analysis is a challenge for ergonomists, because thinking about individual characteristics snaps us out of our usual global view of the work process. I think that is why Céline, Julie, and I kept forgetting to think about gender in the study of cleaners described in chapter 3, and Mélanie and I had the same problem while studying the activity of work-family balancing (chapter 7). In fact, most of the work situations we examine are composed of many workers, and the work processes involve interactions among team members and among teams of workers.

Analyzing work and health in teams

This is a fairly technical point, but I think it is critical for improving work and health. In ergonomics as well as in biology and often even in public health, the unit of analysis is work activity at a specific work station: the workers' individual interactions with their physical, social, and psychological environment. Not very many people are talking about how work teams collectively produce health. Not too many supervisors call their teams in together when it is time for the yearly evaluation, and the annual salary adjustment is not usually collective. In fact, almost the only public reflections I have heard about the gender composition of work teams concern the fact that putting women on boards of directors helps profits.[28]

Ergonomists are starting to think about and analyze how people work together.[29] In many jobs, we need to consider how the different talents, temperaments, and weaknesses can be best meshed together. There has even been a start to thinking about what happens to teamwork when gender-mixed teams organize their work.[30] The more we think in terms of teams, the more we realize that diversity can be good for productivity. But only if management puts some effort into promoting teamwork and protecting the discriminated gender or ethnicity or social class.

I think unions can play an important role in making management aware of the importance of gender relations for good teamwork. Just as solidarity is important for the success of unions, it is important for workers' well-being in general. I think of a bank teller we observed who deplored the bank management's idea of having the tellers compete for who could sell the most mortgages and credit cards. She explained to us that tellers had to work together and consult each other all the time while figuring out how to exchange foreign currency, use a new computer system, treat a difficult customer. Creating competition among tellers was poisoning the atmosphere and hindering the work process.

Comparing women and men

The last technical subject with political importance I want to mention here is a decision scientists make when they compare women's and men's physical performances or physiological assessments. I realized this was important when reading an article related to foot pain during walking.[31] The authors were interested in developing shoes for women and men, so they wanted to compare the pressure on different areas of the sole of the feet while people walked. But what walking speed should be used to compare them? Men are taller than women and take longer steps. So at the same speed, women would be making more steps, and they would be putting pressure on their feet more often.

The authors discussed this problem and decided to use the study participants' "preferred walking speed" to do their measurements. The women's preferred speed turned out to be about the same as the men's, but women, being smaller, had to take 4.4 percent more steps per minute to reach it. When the authors measured the forces on the soles of the participants' feet, they found a lot of other male-female differences. Some of those remaining differences came from the fact that men were generally heavier. Since the difference by sex in the foot-ground interface area is smaller than the weight difference, walking puts more pressure on the parts of men's feet that bear their weight.

This is where the procedure called "normalizing" comes in. The researchers divided the forces on the soles by body weight. This let them compare women's and men's pressure points without being distracted by the differences in weight or in step length. They could then see that women and men exerted force during walking on specific parts of the foot: men toward the heel and toe, women at the arch. They attributed the differences to foot shape and centre of gravity and suggested different shoe designs for women and men.

The procedures of normalizing measurements by body weight and using preferred rather than standard speeds to compare women and men are not always used. Should they be? Is it a good idea to try to make women and men look more alike? Should running performance be compared taking step length, muscle mass, or oxygen metabolism into account, perhaps allowing women and men to compete in the same Olympic events but with different performance assessment methods? Would this solve the problem of how sports competitions can include gender non-conforming women and men?

From a scientific point of view, there is no universal answer to this question; the answer depends on your standpoint. If you want to know how to design new running shoes when the shoes have been previously developed only thinking about men, it is probably a good idea not to normalize, but rather to show all the differences between the (male) population the shoes were designed for and the new (female) population. But if you are interested in equality and want to demonstrate women's capacity to perform some task, it may be better to normalize.

And this is probably true in the workplace. Sometimes, as in designing clothing, tools, and equipment, we want to know all the differences. But other times, it is worth demonstrating that women's performance is similar to men's, given differences in size and shape. And we always want to be careful not to encourage or reify sex or gender stereotypes.

These are political decisions, and they will be taken by the next generation of feminist occupational health scientists.

A research agenda to support working women

It was hard for me to read the posted answers to my questions on ResearchGate about breast size. And just imagine if I had posted a question on ResearchGate about the effects of work on menstrual period pain or menopausal hot flushes! But we really need to know a lot more about women's and men's bodies in the workplace. Here is a very incomplete list of the research that needs to be done if we are to attain health and equality:

> How exactly and to what extent does the size and shape of women's bodies differ from men's, and what are the implications for design of tools, equipment, work spaces, and uniforms? (The need for this information became obvious during the coronavirus pandemic, when women and non-European health care workers complained that their personal protective equipment didn't fit, exposing them to the virus.)

> What is the size and distribution of differences in strength, agility, balance, and endurance between women and men, and what are the implications for design of tasks, tools, training, teamwork, and work schedules? In particular, what are the implications of women's generally lower centre of gravity for lifting techniques?

> In jobs with a physical component, how can teamwork be optimized to benefit from all members' levels of strength, agility, endurance, and balance?

> When women's and men's work activity differs within the same job title, how can health and equality best be protected? Why does activity differ by sex/gender, and should this be allowed, discouraged, or examined closely?

> Why does cold exposure exacerbate menstrual cramps and what could be done about it?[32]

> Are there workplace determinants of urinary incontinence among women and, if so, how should it be prevented? (I can't believe standing at work all day, day after day, doesn't affect the pelvic floor, and it is true that sales and service workers have more incontinence.[33])

> Do men and women have different risks for hand and arm pain related to repetitive work? If so, is it because men and women experience pain and fatigue differently or because they use their muscles differently? How should work be

designed to minimize pain? How can assembly lines be organized to minimize pain for everyone?

> How should data concerning women's and men's physiological characteristics (e.g., walking speed) be analyzed? By comparing men's and women's performances directly or by relating them to the average, median, or maximum for their sex? Or by relating them to height, weight, or muscle dimensions?

> Should health and safety limits on weights lifted at the workplace be different for women and men? for people of different sizes or weights? Should the weight limits be different when the weight is a person who can get aggressive or resist, as in health care or child care? Should people always have machines to help lift weights over a certain limit? the same limit for women and men? How should the shape, texture, and nature of the weights be considered?

> Should the passing level for pre-employment fitness tests (of strength, running speed, agility) differ by gender/sex?[34] Would this favour team building?

> Given the effects of extended work schedules on the body,[35] should pregnancy, nursing, and family responsibilities influence the order of bidding for work schedules in the same way seniority now does? If so, should the number and ages of men's children count the same way as women's?

> How should work breaks be scheduled? Given the domestic responsibilities of many women and their resulting fatigue, should the timing of breaks be more flexible? For example, should it be possible to take more, shorter breaks?

> What kind of scheduling software would help match workers' family responsibilities with available working hours without penalizing other workers?

> What kinds of techniques could help when women enter

previously segregated jobs? Would game-playing help? What should supervisors do? What should happen if a woman refuses to perform a task because of her sex/gender? if a man refuses?

> Should standards for exposure to workplace chemicals be the same for women and men, even when effects can be hormone-related?[36]

We need to promote and reinforce institutions like the Canadian Institute of Gender and Health that support us to do that research, and we need to create and support journals like *New Solutions*, *International Journal of Health Services*, and *American Journal of Industrial Medicine* that will publish the results.

13.
GOING FORWARD TOGETHER

So working women have second-class bodies, second-class jobs, second-class social roles, and are the subject of second-class health research. How should feminists go about improving women's work? How can we eliminate the contradiction between equality and occupational health? What can we do about the shame that is keeping us back? How can we make solidarity work for us?

Changing the employers

Recently one of our research groups had an online meeting about how to design our second intervention with the women's shelters and how to get money for it. On the screen I saw Nathalie Houlfort, a psychology professor, Jessica Riel, an ergonomist and professor of industrial relations, and Vanessa Blanchette-Luong, our (joint) doctoral student. The association of women's shelters had asked us to help them figure out how they could recruit more counsellors. We were open to studying the job as a whole, but we thought we had better concentrate our grant applications on the work-family interface of coordinators and counsellors in the shelters, since the granting organizations would recognize our expertise in work-family interactions. Given the exhausting nature of their work, it was easy to describe challenges to work-family balancing.

But was work-family balancing a problem for the shelter coordinators who managed the schedules? Someone asked Vanessa, who had been observing work in the shelters, how they were handling work-family problems now. She described a series of accommodations—schedule swaps, managers searching for very scarce replacement workers, schedule adjustments. The shelter coordinators did their best to ease the work-family interface, and colleagues did their best to be flexible.

The coordinators invited us to a meeting where they were discussing common problems. Yes, they were jumping through hoops to arrange schedules, trying to accommodate both the more senior counsellors and the young ones with families. One of them said, "I have to work hard on the schedules because if I don't, I'm the one that will end up doing the shift on Sunday night."

I was surprised and impressed. Why? Because we hadn't previously seen so much official good will from managers or dribbling down from employers. Yes, in a study of cleaners, we had seen the occasional sympathetic schedule coordinator who quietly tried to accommodate women with sick children. In retail, sometimes the employer compelled a manager to take a shift if there was no one else to do it. But a manager who was ready to volunteer for a difficult shift? An understanding that managers would make every effort to adjust the schedules to the employee's convenience? No, in the other workplaces, the employers' official attitude seemed to be that any problems with schedules were personal and it was up to the employee to solve them. If you couldn't solve them, you were not competent to hold your job. I couldn't imagine any of the

Transpeq supervisors taking a night shift because a single-parent cleaner couldn't make it. (I asked the union executive and they couldn't imagine it either.) The managers would just threaten to fire the parent, and the parent would have to exert pressure on friends and relatives or leave the child home alone. Even in the face of court decisions that transferred some of the responsibility for the consequences of invasive scheduling to the employer.[1]

More generally, we have not seen many proactive employers of low-paid workers. When women have entered male-dominated jobs in the trades, we haven't observed any particular effort to guide their colleagues in adjusting or to help managers put the teams back together. Admittedly, we probably wouldn't get called in if an employer had succeeded in seamlessly incorporating women. But I have never heard about a situation where they even made an effort, until very recently and under pressure from the government.

Thanks to bad publicity, some employers are being more active about sexual harassment and aggression, especially in well-paid jobs. But acting to moderate everyday exclusion and teasing for factory and service workers? Adjustment of equipment and tools? Attention to the fact that the newly hired women have double the accident rate? Not yet. I often hear of situations where women's accident rates are double men's, without the employers doing anything to help.

What can we do to make the employers evolve? Unions may seem to be an old-fashioned answer, especially now that employers have found all sorts of ways to avoid formally hiring people. As the economy gets Uberized, it has become almost impossible for precarious, sub-contracted workers to join unions. Still, unions are often the only way workers can protect their health. When the workers stick together, they can get change. We have seen a hotel cleaners' union ease their workload, a retail sales union get seats for sales personnel, a cleaners' union desegregate cleaning, a transport union get some recognition for family needs, a teachers' union lower class size, and more.

Government regulation can ease the interface between work and family demands. And when it comes to government policy on employment, solidarity has also paid off. Women's groups in Quebec have joined with the unions to get recognition for family needs, pay equity, and access to employment.

In France, there is now a concerted government effort to train employers and occupational health specialists to fight sexism. And they really, officially call it sexism.[2] A government agency also runs training sessions on women's occupational health for physicians, where there is a firm position that the employers are responsible for adapting their jobs to women. The Quebec and Canadian governments have so far been less proactive.

How can we build solidarity?

Working with others is often difficult. In the transport union, a woman told us she had left her union delegate position because she was under attack from colleagues who held the union responsible for not improving their working conditions. Members often think unions have more power than they really do, and this is hard for union representatives. But it is work that has to be done.

Building solidarity among women, among workers, is hard. Some groups succeed, some don't. Many, many years ago I joined a feminist organization that turned on a group of us, eventually expelling us. I cried a lot at the time. My (professors') union is unusually worker-identified—in a real union confederation that includes cleaners and construction workers. Yet we have swung back and forth between excluding other university employees and solidarity with them, between a narrow economic agenda and social justice concerns. The feminist movement I support is now licking its wounds from a painful split over (to simplify it) women's "agency" with regard to hijabs, sex work, and gender fluidity. Our choices oscillate between collective and individual concerns.

Political fights are hard to take, and building CINBIOSE has involved its share of suffering. My former students remind me that there was a time when most of our young men left CINBIOSE after discussions about the place of men in the feminist movement. Building refuges sometimes seems to mean building walls, and we have to struggle to figure out where to put the doors. But it is worth the struggle.

Overcoming shame

Writing this book, I have had my own times of feeling ashamed of my interventions. For example: questioning our methods and results led to a scientific article I published in 2017 about the cleaners described in chapter 3,[3] the one describing how merging the "light" and "heavy" work categories ended up with fewer women and no real gains in health for the women who remained. I entitled the article "A feminist intervention that hurt women" (without a question mark) because I was feeling guilty toward all the older women cleaners I had met, the ones who had left their jobs. These poor women had been forced out of their economic niche because of my feminist ideology. How unthinking was that? I started this book as a wakeup call to feminists to make sure we did our interventions more carefully. As in chapters 6 and 7, I was going to examine how Nicole's and my teams differ in approach and how our approaches have led each of us to fail to a certain extent.

But, ten years after we finished our study of cleaners, when my colleagues questioned the union representatives about the interventions in hospital cleaning, they said the intervention had been a success—we had succeeded in destroying a female ghetto, we had helped get more money for the women, we had taught everyone about the importance of "light" work, and we had gotten management to implement a fair number of improvements in the cleaning jobs. Yes, we probably could have done more to push the employer to adapt the job for women. And I should have listened more to the cleaners. But maybe we have to think in terms of baby steps—desegregation may have been a good step on the way to empowerment of women. And shame may have kept me from exploring more ways I could have helped.

Facing down the dragon

Analyzing how we have intervened in the past, Marie Laberge and the other CINBIOSE researchers have divided our interventions into three types: those where sex/gender was made an explicit part of the intervention, those where sex/gender analysis was implicit but not articulated, and those without a sex/gender analysis.[4] The existence of this last category surprised us. How was it possible that people we trained had stayed unconscious of gender throughout their interventions? I remember particularly a young woman who presented a seminar on her work with the same gardeners' union I mentioned at the beginning of chapter 4, where tasks were informally organized by gender and where equipment was not adapted for women. Almost thirty years after our study, she duly noted that half the workers were (still) women but never mentioned sex or gender during her work analysis. At the end, I asked her whether the women and the men she observed were doing the same tasks. She replied that they must have been because there were half women. A meaningless answer. I knew that, just a few months before, ergonomist Marie Laberge had trained that speaker in how to apply sex/gender analyses to her interventions. But she had clearly not used the training. Why?

We shouldn't underestimate how hard it is to take on gender issues in the workplace, and how uncomfortable it makes us feel. To some of us, it seems inappropriate to introduce a "political" issue during an academic or professional project. Others, empathetic toward the workers, feel awkward bringing up a subject we think workers don't want to hear about and that might start quarrels. Some are afraid that managers will react by barring them from the workplace, thus making it impossible for them to improve the work environment. And many ergonomists find it inappropriate to push in an area no one has been complaining about—we are supposed to listen to the workplace and then decide how to help make it better, not advance our own agenda. It's not like there aren't enough visible musculoskeletal disorders to deal with in these workplaces.

In the end, I don't think we can decide once and for all to take either Nicole's or my own approach to transforming workplaces. Sometimes, naming gender is a distraction that turns worker against worker and blocks progress in improving work for everyone. Sometimes, naming gender can lead management, union, or government officials to understand and deal with an injustice. Sometimes, as with the communications technicians, naming gender is absolutely necessary to help women articulate their suffering and give them the energy to get together and fight back, or to allow them to concede defeat and pursue their battle elsewhere. Probably the most important element in both Nicole's and my research teams is that all of us are conscious of sex/gender issues and want to work toward gender equality and better working conditions for women.

Sticking together despite opposition

My colleagues and I would not have survived in academia without our research centre, CINBIOSE, and the many women who have given their scarce time and energy to keeping it alive. It has not been easy; opposition within the university has at times become relentless—and right now is one of those times. I didn't understand why our colleagues in the science faculty kept trying to close CINBIOSE down until one day I was asked to meet with a colleague from another science department, whom I will call Michel.

We were trying to figure out how to reorganize a particularly troublesome methods course that was alternately trying to cover too much and too little. After we had been conversing for an hour or so, Michel asked me, apropos of nothing, "Aren't you the director of CINBIOSE?" I said yes. "But, but . . ." he said, and trailed off. "But what?" I asked. And finally he came out with it—he had suddenly realized we had been talking in a "normal" (his expression) way for a long time, despite my association with a group of raging feminists who didn't give a hoot for science (my summary of his halting description). And our subsequent exchange made me understand why many of the students in my methods course had been making trouble. A group of powerful men in the program had convinced themselves, Michel, and many students that we were a danger to quality education and scientific research.

Michel had no particular examples of our unworthiness to offer (and he was pretty embarrassed even to be talking with me about it), but he left our meeting only fractionally less frightened of CINBIOSE. I understood that it was just our solidarity, and the respect of a very few men and women in high places, that was protecting us from closure. What were they so afraid of? Three things, I think. The university is still fairly young as universities go and its science faculty had still to prove itself as competent as the competition. It hasn't decided whether to be a second-class version of the older universities or, more scarily, to branch out in new directions. CINBIOSE, with its emphasis on community-oriented research in environmental and occupational health, could appear to them to be turning its back on conventional, laboratory, "evidence-based" science and thus on academic recognition and prestige.

CINBIOSE was also not kosher in that many of our researchers came from the social sciences and even the arts. To many of my biology department colleagues, these were not scientists, so what were they doing in the science faculty, weakening our image?

And finally, Michel's hesitant language made it obvious that the men found our style obnoxious and scary. We were noisier and more explicit about their power games than a bunch of women had any right to be. (Answer number one: we are a multidisciplinary research centre, which is something universities are supposed to be supporting. Answer number two: we have been very successful getting research grants together for over thirty years, which universities are supposed to respect.)

But the bottom line is that CINBIOSE has succeeded in creating a safe space, despite the Michels and their pals. Creating safe spaces for women is worth the effort it requires to confront the opposition. Setting up women's committees in unions, women's caucuses in government, and women's organizations generally is a way to fight the dragon.

We need to promote solidarity with women who are not necessarily just like us

The links among CINBIOSE researchers are strong, but they would not have been enough to save our centre and our orientation, at least temporarily, without the support and solidarity we have received from the union women's committees and union health and safety advocates. Our partnerships with women and men in the unions have educated and inspired us. In Quebec, we are lucky enough to have a union movement whose women's services can regularly collaborate with feminist movements involved in improving women's work, so we have also been able to work with and learn from women's groups and from broad coalitions of women workers.

My university, ambivalent as it has always been about science that responds to community priorities rather than those of companies or scientific institutions, has nevertheless continued to support the efforts of its community outreach service to keep university science within the reach of the Quebec citizens who pay for it. It is really, really too bad that, after forty years, we are still the only university in Canada that provides funds, personnel, released time for professors, and official recognition for community-initiated collaborative research and training. And it is not because we haven't tried to make the model known. Any university employees or community organizations reading this can contact me (at messing.karen@uqam.ca) and I will explain how it is set up and all the protections for researchers and for the community organizations.

Facing the paradoxes

I started to write this book because I saw that working women were being hurt by our understandable feminist wish to underplay biological differences between the sexes that impact women's performance and well-being in the workplace. I wanted workplaces to accept their responsibility to adapt to our bodies as they are, whether or not we can make ourselves stronger. I want to learn more about our physiological advantages—better endurance? more stability?—so that work teams can profit from them.

During the writing I have realized that we are all being hurt by denial of the social roles imposed on or even chosen by women, men, and everyone else. I want workplaces to adapt to all the caring responsibilities women are now assuming, whether or not men should be sharing them more. I want people to be able to express whatever gender-associated identities they have, without feeling they need to apologize or conceal them. And we all need to get together, stop being ashamed of our bodies and our conditioning, and fight for equality and health. Come join us.

ACKNOWLEDGEMENTS

I want to thank the many people who helped me write this book. Jessica Riel read and commented on an early version, helping me understand the connections between what we do and the feminist movement. Mélanie Lefrançois and Valérie Lederer gave me useful detailed comments. Julie Côté and Fabienne Goutille gave me new ideas. Marie Laberge, Mathieu-Joël Gervais, and Marie-Eve Major passed on several very useful criticisms. Eliane Kinsley read and commented on many versions from her perspective as a writer and a woman in the trades.

Mahée Gilbert-Ouimet made helpful suggestions about chapter 12 but she isn't responsible for any errors.

Susan Braedley very kindly organized a discussion of the manuscript among her amazing students at Carleton. Janna Klostermann, Prince Owusu, Christine Streeter, Lauren Brooks-Cleator, and Tara MacWhinney provided lots of helpful and stimulating suggestions, many of which I tried to follow.

Barbara Scales, Eliane Kinsley, Mikail Al-Aidroos, and Sheila Santos helped me get started. Daood Aidroos pointed out that I have emotions about the experiences I had in the workplace and that I should admit it.

The whole GESTE (Genre, Équité, Santé, Travail, Environnement) team, led by Marie Laberge and supported by the Institute of Gender and Health of the Canadian Institutes of Health Research (grant number #153 464), stimulated and pushed me deeper and deeper into thinking about how we could do better (and how we were not doing so badly); some of our results are presented in chapters 6 and 7. Especially thank you to the Activité 3 team: Marie Laberge, Mélanie Lefrançois, Hélène Sultan-Taïeb, Jessica Riel, and Mathieu-Joël Gervais, and our partners Relais-femmes and Femmes et environnement. I also acknowledge the help and support of the SAGE research team led by Jessica Riel and financed by the Fonds de recherche du Québec—Société et culture, as well as the work/family articulation research group led by Nathalie Houlfort and financed by the Social Science and Humanities Research Council of Canada.

Thanks also to the Service aux collectivités of the Université du Québec à Montréal for support, guidance, and help over many years (Sylvie de Grosbois, Martine Blanc, Eve Marie Lampron).

I am indebted to the people who pulled me through two months of hospitalization and four months of rehab after my bicycle accident, with my morale and body almost intact: my family (Messings, Al-Aidrooses, Sormanys, Santoses), and "the gang": Ana Maria Seifert, Jessica Riel, Mélanie Lefrançois, Marie Laberge, Hélène Sultan-Taïeb, Eve Laperrière, Martin Chadoin, as well as Ellen Balka, Cathy Vaillancourt, Johanne Saint-Charles, France Tissot, Johanne Leduc, Gilles Blais, Micheline Cyr, Donna Mergler, Susan Stock, Yolande Cohen, Stéphane Desjardins, Pierre D'Amour, Julie Côté, Marie-Eve Major, Vanessa Blanchette-Luong, Katherine Lippel, Norman King, and Christian Dufour. Not to mention the incredibly generous medical and nursing staff at Clifford Hospital,

Guangzhou, and my physiotherapists Julie Gardiner and Vincent Sigouin.

Thank you so much to the union movement for your help in educating me, especially the women's committees and Micheline Boucher, Gisèle Bourret, Claudette Carbonneau, Lucie Dagenais, Ghislaine Fleury, Carole Gingras, Danièle Hébert, Pierre Lefebvre, the late Nicole Lepage, and Chantal Locat.

I am grateful to the people at Between the Lines, particularly the always-stimulating and so very patient editor Amanda Crocker, the meticulous and resourceful Tilman Lewis, the helpful Devin Clancy. Thanks so much to Karina Palmitesta for the title idea. And, for the French translation, to the helpful people at Écosociété: David Murray, Élodie Comtois, and the hardworking and persistent Sylvain Neault. And a special thanks to Inah Kim, Kyu Yeon Kim, Sae Eun Kim, Hyeon Seouk Lee, and Min Choi for translating *Pain and Prejudice* as a labour of love, and who with Hyunjoo Kim have worked so hard to advance working women's issues in South Korea.

I owe and intellectual and emotional debt to inspiring authors Linda Tirado (*Hand to Mouth: Living in Bootstrap America*) and Caroline Criado Perez (*Invisible Women: Exposing Data Bias in a World Designed for Men*) and to Pat Armstrong, who has written too many books to count and come up with too many ideas to cite.

What to say about Pierre Sormany, an expert editor and an infinitely generous partner? From the beginning Pierre made countless helpful suggestions and then consoled me when I got overwhelmed by them. Merci énormément, je t'aime à la folie.

Thanks to all the courageous women who started the #MeToo movement and named what so many of us feel. And to all the valiant women workers who inspired me.

NOTES

Preface

1 Kari Bø, Raul Artal, Ruben Barakat, et al., "Exercise and Pregnancy in Recreational and Elite Athletes: 2016 Evidence Summary from the IOC Expert Group Meeting, Lausanne. Part 1—Exercise in Women Planning Pregnancy and Those Who Are Pregnant," *British Journal of Sports Medicine* 50,10 (2016), 571–89, doi: 10.1136/bjsports-2016-096218.

2 Karen Messing, *Pain and Prejudice: What Science Can Learn about Work from the People Who Do It* (Toronto: Between the Lines, 2014), preface and chapter 1.

3 *À notre santé,* co-produced by Dominique Barbier, Josiane Jouet, and Louise Vandelac.

4 Stephanie Premji, Karen Messing, and Katherine Lippel, "Broken English, Broken Bones?: Mechanisms Linking Language Proficiency and Occupational Health in a Montreal Garment Factory," *International Journal of Health Services* 38,1 (2008), 1–19.

5 Stephanie Premji, "Immigrant Men and Women's Occupational Health: Questioning the Myths," in *Sick and Tired: Health and Safety Inequalities*, ed. Stephanie Premji (Black Point, NS: Fernwood Publishing, 2018), 105–116.

1. The third hour

1 Lena Gonäs, Anders Wikman, Marjan Vaez, et al., "Gender Segregation of Occupations and Sustainable Employment: A Prospective Population-Based Cohort Study," *Scandinavian Journal of Public Health* 47,3 (2019), 348–356, doi: 10.1177/1403494818785255.

2 All names appearing in this book have been changed, in accordance with our ethics procedures, unless a surname is included.

3 Marie-Christine Thibault, "Les conditions d'insertion et de maintien des femmes dans les emplois non-traditionnels : l'impact des outils et des équipements de travail," MSc thesis, Université du Québec à Montréal, 2004.

4 From an interview transcript:
Je ne sais pas qu'est-ce qui a provoqué ça. Le technicien en face de moi, en parlant à la serveuse : « Maudite bitch! », des affaires de même. Moi ça a été : « Pardon! », là j'ai regardé la serveuse et j'ai dit : «Excuse là, mais moi je ne servirais pas du monde qui me parle de même ». (Le technicien a répondu) « Ah! C'est en joke! Tu devrais te tenir avec nous autres les gars! » J'ai dit : « Je regrette mais ça, ça s'appelle du savoir-vivre, s'adresser à quelqu'un comme ça, je trouve absolument pas ça drôle, mais pas pantoute! » Ils se sont tous levés d'un coup! Je te jure on était 10 à la table! « Oui, ok, c'est correct! Je pense qu'on va y aller! » Ils sont tous partis, j'ai fini mes toasts toute seule! (Sophie)

5 Karen Messing, Ana Maria Seifert, and Vanessa Couture, "Les femmes dans les métiers non-traditionnels : Le général, le particulier et l'ergonomie," *Travailler* 15 (2006), 131–48.

6 Katelyn F. Allison, Karen A. Keenan, Timothy C Sell, et al., "Musculoskeletal, Biomechanical, and Physiological Gender Differences in the US Military," *US Army Medical Department Journal* (Apr–Jun 2015), 22–32.

7 Patrick Duguay, Alexandre Boucher, Pascale Prud'homme, et al., *Lésions professionnelles indemnisées au Québec en 2010–2012. Profil statistique par industrie—catégorie Professionnelle.* Report R-963 (Montreal: Institut de recherche Robert-Sauvé en Santé et en Sécurité du Travail, Montreal, 2017).

8 Oyebode A. Taiwo, Linda F. Cantley, Martin D. Slade, et al., "Sex Differences in Injury Patterns among Workers in Heavy

Manufacturing," *American Journal of Epidemiology* 169,2 (2009), 161–6, doi: 10.1093/aje/kwn304.

9   Sophie Brochu, "Sophie Brochu : L'authenticité et la passion au service de la société," interview by Marie-France Bazzo, *Les grands entretiens*, Radio-Canada, December 6, 2016, https://ici.radio-canada.ca.

10   Commission des droits de la personne et droits de la jeunesse, "La commission des droits de la personne et des droits de la jeunesse se réjouit du jugement rendu par la Cour d'appel dans l'affaire Gaz Metro," June 30, 2011, www.cdpdj.qc.ca.

11   Éducation et Enseignement supérieur Québec, "Métiers et professions traditionnellement masculins," www.education.gouv.qc.ca.

12   https://cinbiose.uqam.ca; Messing, *Pain and Prejudice*, chapter 8.

13   Marie Laberge, Vanessa Luong-Blanchette, Arnaud Blanchard, et al., "Impacts of Considering Sex and Gender during Intervention Studies in Occupational Health: Researchers' Perspectives," *Applied Ergonomics* 82, doi: j.apergo.2019.102960.

2. Shame and silence in health care

1   Confédération des syndicats nationaux, "Une syndicaliste récompensée par le Lieutenant-gouverneur," May 7, 2012, www.csn.qc.ca.

2   The training program was part of my teaching load as a university professor, thanks to the agreement between my university and the three major union confederations in Quebec.

3   François Aubry and Isabelle Feillou, "Une forme de gestion désincarnée de l'activité," *Perspectives interdisciplinaires sur le travail et la santé* 21,1 (2019), doi: 10.4000/pistes.6177.

4   François Aubry, "Les raisons du manque d'attrait du métier de préposée aux bénéficiaires," *Le Devoir,* February 26, 2018, www.ledevoir.com; Esther Cloutier and Patrice Duguay, "Impact de l'avance en age sur les scenarios d'accidents et les indicateurs de lesions dans le secteur de la sante et des services sociaux" (Montreal: Institut Robert-Sauvé de Recherche en Santé et en Sécurité du Travail, 1996), vol. 1, ch. 5 and Table 6-6; Hasanat Alamgir, Yuri Cvitkovich, Shicheng Yu, and Annalee Yassi, "Work-Related Injury among Direct Care Occupations in British Columbia, Canada," *Occupational Medicine* 64 (2007), 769–75.

5   Sylvie Bédard, "L'importance des TMS chez les soignants en quelques chiffres," *Objectif Prévention* 39,2 (2016), 19.

6   Ontario Health Coalition, *Caring in Crisis: Ontario's Long-Term Care PSW Shortage* (Toronto: Ontario Health Coalition, 2019), www.ontariohealthcoalition.ca.

7   Cloutier and Duguay, "Impact de l'avance en age."

8   Karen Messing and Diane Elabidi, "Desegregation and Occupational Health: How Male and Female Hospital Attendants Collaborate on Work Tasks Requiring Physical Effort," *Policy and Practice in Health and Safety* 1 (2003), 83–103.

9   Messing and Elabidi, "Desegregation and Occupational Health."

10 Karen Messing, *One-Eyed Science: Occupational Health and Working Women* (Philadelphia: Temple University Press, 1998).

11 Monique Lortie, "Structural Analysis of Occupational Accidents Affecting Orderlies in a Geriatric Hospital," *Journal of Occupational Medicine* 29 (1987), 437–44.

3. A feminist intervention that hurt women?

1   Some of the material in this chapter was originally published as a scientific article: Karen Messing, "A Feminist Intervention That Hurt Women: Biological Differences, Ergonomics and Occupational Health," *New Solutions: A Journal of Occupational and Environmental Health Policy* 27,3 (2017), 304–318. I have described the technical and social challenges to cleaners, ignored or treated with contempt by those around them, in *Pain and Prejudice*, chapter 2. The economic arguments against subcontracting cleaning work are given in Shimaa Elkomy, Graham Cookson, and Simon Jones, "Cheap and Dirty: The Effect of Contracting Out Cleaning on Efficiency and Effectiveness," *Public Administration Review* 79,2 (2019), 193–202.

2   Not the hospitals' real names.

3   Until very recently, any mention of sex and gender in relation to health was sufficient to classify research as social science, and even now, my ergonomics research is often referred to by journalists and even some academics as sociology, a field I know little about.

4   Then a graduate student, Céline Chatigny later became a professor and collaborated in other studies such as those described in chapters 1 and 8.

5   Karen Messing, Céline Chatigny, and Julie Courville, "'Light' and
     'Heavy' Work in the Housekeeping Service of a Hospital," *Applied
     Ergonomics* 29 (1998), 451–59.

6   Sarah J. Locke, Joanne S Colt, Patricia A. Stewart, et al., "Identifying
     Gender Differences in Reported Occupational Information from
     Three U.S. Population-Based Case-Control Studies," *Occupational
     and Environmental Medicine* 71,12 (2014), 855–64, doi: 10.1136/
     oemed-2013-101801.

7   Messing, Chatigny, and Courville, "'Light' and 'Heavy' Work"; Karen
     Messing, "Hospital Trash: Cleaners Speak of Their Role in Disease
     Prevention," *Medical Anthropology Quarterly* 12 (1998), 168–87.

8   No comparison could be done for South Hospital, since we had no
     data from the earlier time.

9   Bénédicte Calvet, Jessica Riel, Vanessa Couture, and Karen Messing,
     "Work Organisation and Gender among Hospital Cleaners in
     Quebec after the Merger of 'Light' and 'Heavy' Work Classifications,"
     Ergonomics 55 (2012), 160–72, doi: 10.1080/00140139.2011.576776.

10   Confédération des Syndicats Nationaux, *Ciel, un hippopotame dans
     mon milieu de travail : Guide de sensibilisation aux impacts sur la santé au
     travail de rapports hommes-femmes difficiles* (Montreal: Confédération
     des Syndicats Nationaux, May 2005), www.csn.qc.ca.

4. Jobs and bodies

1   Karen Messing, Lucie Dumais, Julie Courville, et al., "Evaluation
     of Exposure Data from Men and Women with the Same Job Title,"
     Journal of Occupational Medicine 36,8 (1994), 913–17.

2   Statistics Canada, Portrait of Canada's Labour Force, "Table 2. The
     20 most common occupations among women aged 15 years and
     over and the share of women in the total workforce, May 2011,"
     www.statcan.gc.ca.

3   Eve Laperrière, Karen Messing, and Renée Bourbonnais, "Work
     Activity in Food Service: The Significance of Customer Relations,
     Tipping Practices and Gender for Preventing Musculoskeletal
     Disorders," *Applied Ergonomics* 58 (2017), 89–101.

4   « Dans ma tête, je me répète : verre d'eau / facture / ketchup / café-thé
     / verre d'eau / facture / ketchup / café-thé … »

5   Eve Laperrière, "Etude du travail de serveuses de restaurant," PhD diss., Université du Québec à Montréal, 2014.

6   Lynnelle K. Smith, Jennifer L. Lelas, and D. Casey Kerrigan, "Gender Differences in Pelvic Motions and Center of Mass Displacement during Walking: Stereotypes Quantified," *Journal of Women's Health & Gender-Based Medicine* 11,5 (2002), 453–58; Magdalena I. Tolea, Paul T. Costa, Antonio Terracciano, et al., "Sex-Specific Correlates of Walking Speed in a Wide Age-Ranged Population," *Journals of Gerontology: Psychological Science and Social Science* 65B,2 (2010), 174–84.

7   Laperrière, Messing, and Bourbonnais, "Work Activity in Food Service."

8   Matthew Parrett, "Customer Discrimination in Restaurants: Dining Frequency Matters," *Journal of Labor Research* 32,2 (2011), 87–112.

9   Laperrière, Messing, and Bourbonnais, "Work Activity in Food Service."

10 Lucie Dumais, Karen Messing, Ana Maria Seifert, et al., "Make Me a Cake as Fast as You Can: Determinants of Inertia and Change in the Sexual Division of Labour of an Industrial Bakery," *Work, Employment and Society* 7,3 (1993), 363–82.

11 Aude Lacourt, France Labrèche, Mark S. Goldberg, et al., "Agreement in Occupational Exposures between Men and Women Using Retrospective Assessments by Expert Coders," *Annals of Work Exposure and Health* 62,9 (2018), 1159–70.

12 Amanda Eng, Andrea 't Mannetje, Dave McLean, et al., "Gender Differences in Occupational Exposure Patterns," *Occupational and Environmental Medicine* 68,12 (2011), 888–94.

13 Nicole Vézina and Julie Courville, "Integration of Women into Traditionally Masculine Jobs," *Women and Health* 18,3 (1992), 97–118.

14 Donna Mergler, Carole Brabant, Nicole Vézina, and Karen Messing, "The Weaker Sex?: Men in Women's Working Conditions Report Similar Health Symptoms," *Journal of Occupational Medicine* 29,5 (1987), 417–21; Messing, Chatigny, and Courville, "'Light' and 'Heavy' Work."

15 Laurent Vogel, *Women and Occupational Diseases: The Case of Belgium* (Brussels: European Trade Union Institute, 2011), 40, www.etui.org.

16 France Tissot, Karen Messing, and Susan R. Stock, "Standing, Sitting

and Associated Working Conditions in the Quebec Population in 1998," *Ergonomics* 48,3 (2005), 249–69.

17 Messing, Chatigny, and Courville, "'Light' and 'Heavy' Work."

18 Luc Cloutier-Villeneuve, "Heures travaillées au Québec, aux États-Unis et ailleurs au Canada en 2017," *Travail et Rémunération* 13 (2019), 1–24, https://stat.gouv.qc.ca.

19 Melissa Moyser and Amanda Burlock, "Time Use: Total Work Burden, Unpaid Work, and Leisure" (Ottawa: Statistics Canada, 2018), Chart 3, www.statcan.gc.ca.

20 Calculated from Frank D. Denton and Sylvia Ostry, *Relevés chronologiques de la main-d'œuvre canadienne* (Ottawa: Statistics Canada, 1967), 26, http://publications.gc.ca.

21 Calculated from Statistics Canada, "Labour Force Characteristics by Province, Monthly, Unadjusted for Seasonality" (Ottawa: Statistics Canada, 2020), www.statcan.gc.ca.

22 Statistics Canada, "Labour in Canada: Key Results from the 2016 Census," Chart 9 (Ottawa: Statistics Canada, 2017), www.statcan.gc.ca.

23 Michael Baker and Kirsten Cornelson, "Gender Based Occupational Segregation and Sex Differences in Sensory, Motor and Spatial Aptitudes" (Toronto:University of Toronto, 2016), https://econ.sites.olt.ubc.ca.

24 Alexis Riopel, Guillaume Levasseur, Cédric Gagnon, and Antoine Béland, "Les professions à risque sont-elles plus occupées par des femmes?," *Le Devoir*, May 8, 2020, www.ledevoir.com.

25 Campbell Robertson and Robert Gebeloff, "How Millions of Women Became the Most Essential Workers in America," *New York Times* (April 18, 2020).

26 Sharanjit Uppal and Sébastien LaRochelle-Côté, "Changes in the Occupational Profile of Young Men and Women in Canada" (Ottawa: Statistics Canada, 2014), www.statcan.gc.ca.

27 Florence Chappert, Karen Messing, Eric Peltier, and Jessica Riel, "Conditions de travail et parcours dans l'entreprise : vers une transformation qui intègre l'ergonomie et le genre?," *Revue multidisciplinaire sur l'emploi, le syndicalisme et le travail* (REMEST) 9,2 (2014), 46–67, www.erudit.org; Florence Chappert and Laurence Théry, "Égalité entre les femmes et les hommes et santé au travail," *Perspectives interdisciplinaires sur le travail et la santé* 18,2 (2016), 1–28,

http://journals.openedition.org; Florence Chappert, "Gendered Indicators in OHS: A Number to Convince and Transform Public Policies," in *Proceedings of the 20th Congress of the International Ergonomics Association* IX (Florence, Italy: International Ergonomics Association, 2018), 354–62.

28 Chappert, Messing, Peltier, and Riel, "Conditions de travail et parcours dans l'entreprise."

5. Same, different, or understudied?

1 Kristin W. Springer, Jeanne Mager Stellman, and Rebecca Jordan-Young, "Beyond a Catalogue of Differences: A Theoretical Frame and Good Practice Guidelines for Researching Sex/Gender in Human Health," *Social Science & Medicine* 74,11 (2012), 1817–24.

2 See also the discussion of continuous variation vs. bimodality in Anne Fausto-Sterling, "On the Critiques of the Concept of Sex: An Interview with Anne Fausto-Sterling," *Differences: A Journal of Feminist Cultural Studies* 27,1 (2016), 189–205.

3 Michael I. Greenberg, John A. Curtis, and David Vearrier, "The Perception of Odor Is Not a Surrogate Marker for Chemical Exposure: A Review of Factors Influencing Human Odor Perception," *Clinical Toxicology* 51,2 (2013), 70–76, doi: 10.3109/15563650.2013.767908.

4 Stavros Sifakis, Vasilis Androutsopoulos, Aristeidis M. Tsatsakis, and Demetrios A. Spandidos, "Human Exposure to Endocrine Disrupting Chemicals: Effects on the Male and Female Reproductive Systems," *Environmental Toxicology and Pharmacology* 51 (April 2017), 56–70, doi: 10.1016/j.etap.2017.02.024.

5 I am allowed to explain genetics because I taught it for many years; in fact, my PhD is in genetics and I only got trained in ergonomics fifteen years later. See chapter 1 of my 2014 book *Pain and Prejudice*.

6 Anne Fausto-Sterling, "Beyond Difference: A Biologist's Perspective," *Journal of Social Issues* 53,2 (1997), 233–58; Anne Fausto-Sterling, "Against Dichotomy," *Evolutionary Studies in Imaginative Culture* 1,1 (2017), 63–65. And see also her comments at Anne Fausto-Sterling, "Why Sex Is Not Binary," *New York Times*, opinion, Oct. 25, 2018, www.nytimes.com.

7   Springer, Stellman, and Jordan-Young, "Beyond a Catalogue of Differences."

8   Almost always women—some exceptional people (Klinefelter's syndrome) with two or more X chromosomes and a Y chromosome look like men. And of course, some people classed chromosomally as men define themselves as women or non-binary or undergo transformation using chemicals or surgery, just as some people classified chromosomally as men define themselves otherwise.

9   Zohreh Jangravi, Mehdi Alikhani, Babak Arefnezhad, et al., "A Fresh Look at the Male-Specific Region of the Human Y Chromosome," *Journal of Proteome Research* 12,1 (2013), 6–22.

10 Nichole Rigby and Rob J. Kulathinal, "Genetic Architecture of Sexual Dimorphism in Humans," *Journal of Cellular Physiology* 230,10 (2015), 2304–2310.

11 Ruth Hubbard and Anne Fausto-Stirling have written about this in detail. See also the blog of Harvard University's GenderSci Lab at www.genderscilab.org/blog.

12 See for example Jason Pham, "Serena Williams Shut Down Body Critics: 'I Am Strong and Muscular—and Beautiful,'" *Business Insider*, May 2018, www.businessinsider.com.

13 Allan Keefe and Harry Angel, *2012 Canadian Forces Anthropometric Survey (CFAS) Final Report* (Ottawa: Defence Research and Development Canada, 2015).

14 Kalypso Karastergiou, Steven R. Smith, Andrew S. Greenberg, and Susan K. Fried, "Sex Differences in Human Adipose Tissues—The Biology of Pear Shape," *Biology of Sex Differences* 3,1 (2012), 13.

15 M.D. Tillman, J.A. Bauer, J.H. Cauraugh, and M.H. Trimble, "Differences in Lower Extremity Alignment between Males and Females: Potential Predisposing Factors for Knee Injury," *Journal of Sports Medicine and Physical Fitness* 45,3 (2005), 355–59.

16 Hana Brzobohatá, Vaclav Krajíček, Zdenek Horák, and Jana Velemínská, "Sexual Dimorphism of the Human Tibia through Time: Insights into Shape Variation Using a Surface-Based Approach," *PLoS One* 11,11 (2016), e0166461, doi: 10.1371/journal.pone.0166461.

17 Inga Krauss, Stefan Grau, Marlene Mauch, et al., "Sex-Related Differences in Foot Shape," *Ergonomics* 51,11 (2008), 1693–1709.

18 Yoram Epstein, Chen Fleischmann, Ran Yanovich, and Yuval Heled, "Physiological and Medical Aspects That Put Women Soldiers

at Increased Risk for Overuse Injuries," *Journal of Strength and Conditioning Research* 29,11 suppl. (2015), S107–10.

19   André Plamondon, Denys Denis, Christian Larivière, et al., *Biomechanics and Ergonomics in Women Material Handlers,* report R808 (Montreal: Institut de recherche Robert-Sauvé en santé et en sécurité du travail du Québec, 2008).

20   Jason Bouffard, Romain Martinez, André Plamondon, et al., "Sex Differences in Glenohumeral Muscle Activation and Coactivation during a Box Lifting Task," *Ergonomics* 62,7 (2019), 1–12, doi: 10.1080/00140139.2019.1640396.

21   Romain Martinez, Jason Bouffard, Benjamin Michaud, et al., "Sex Differences in Upper Limb 3D Joint Contributions during a Lifting Task," *Ergonomics* 62,5 (2019), 682–93, doi: 10.1080/00140139.2019.1571245.

22   Yoram Epstein, Ran Yanovich, D.S. Moran, and Yuval Heled, "Physiological Employment Standards IV: Integration of Women in Combat Units—Physiological and Medical Considerations," *European Journal of Applied Physiology* 113,11 (2013), 2673–90, doi: 10.1007/s00421-012-2558-7.

23   K.M. Haizlip, B.C. Harrison, and L.A. Leinwand, "Sex-Based Differences in Skeletal Muscle Kinetics and Fiber-Type Composition (Review)," *Physiology* 30,1 (2015), 30–39, doi: 10.1152/physiol.00024.2014.

24   Gregory Martel, Stephen Roth, Frederick M. Ivey, et al., "Age and Sex Affect Human Muscle Fibre Adaptations to Heavy-Resistance Strength Training," *Experimental Physiology* 91,2 (2006), 457–64.

25   Sandra K. Hunter, "Sex Differences in Human Fatigability: Mechanisms and Insight to Physiological Responses," *Acta Physiologica (Oxford)* 210,4 (2014), 768–89.

26   Amber Dance, "Genes That Escape Silencing on the Second X Chromosome May Drive Disease," *The Scientist*, March 1, 2020, www.the-scientist.com.

27   Larissa Fedorowich, Kim Emery, Bridget Gervasi, and Julie N. Côté, "Gender Differences in Neck/Shoulder Muscular Patterns in Response to Repetitive Motion Induced Fatigue," *Journal of Electromyography and Kinesiology* 23,5 (2013), 1183–9, doi: 10.1016/j.jelekin.2013.06.005.

28   Kim Emery and Julie N. Côté, "Repetitive Arm Motion-Induced

Fatigue Affects Shoulder but Not Endpoint Position Sense,"
Experimental Brain Research 216,4 (2012), 553–64. doi: 10.1007/
s00221-011-2959-6.

29 A clear and understandable review of her work on sex differences
in muscular strength can be found on Youtube: Julie Côté,
"Can Using a Sex/Gender Lens Provide New Insights into MSD
Mechanisms?," keynote presentation at PREMUS 2016, Toronto,
https://youtu.be/8sd4ei8VuFU.

30 Bouffard, Martinez, Plamondon, et al., "Sex Differences in
Glenohumeral Muscle Activation and Coactivation"; Martinez,
Bouffard, Michaud, et al., "Sex Differences in Upper Limb 3D Joint
Contributions"; Denis Gagnon, André Plamondon, and Christian
Larivière, "A Comparison of Lumbar Spine and Muscle Loading
between Male and Female Workers during Box Transfers," *Journal
of Biomechanics* 81 (2018), 76–85, doi: 10.1016/j.jbiomech.2018.09.017;
André Plamondon, Christian Larivière, Denys Denis, et al.,
"Difference between Male and Female Workers Lifting the Same
Relative Load when Palletizing Boxes," *Applied Ergonomics* 60 (2017),
93–102, doi: 10.1016/j.apergo.2016.10.014.

31 Lena Karlqvist, Ola Leijon, and Annika Harenstäm, "Physical
Demands in Working Life and Individual Physical Capacity,"
European Journal of Applied Physiology 89,6 (2003), 536–47.

32 Joan M. Stevenson, D.R. Greenhorn, John Timothy Bryant, et al.,
"Gender Differences in Performance of a Selection Test Using the
Incremental Lifting Machine," *Applied Ergonomics* 27,1 (1996), 45–52.

33 Katherine Lippel, "Preventive Reassignment of Pregnant or Breast-
Feeding Workers: The Québec Model," *New Solutions: A Journal of
Occupational and Environmental Health Policy* 8,2 (1998), 267–80.

34 Anne-Renée Gravel, Jessica Riel, and Karen Messing, "Protecting
Pregnant Workers while Fighting Sexism: Work-Pregnancy Balance
and Pregnant Nurses' Resistance in Québec Hospitals," *New Solutions:
A Journal of Occupational and Environmental Health Policy* 27,3 (2017),
424–37.

35 Stéphane Crespo, "L'emploi du temps professionnel et domestique
des personnes agees de 15 ans et plus," *Coup d'œil sociodémographique*
[online] 62 (Quebec: Institut de la statistique du Québec, March
2018), 1–10, www.stat.gouv. qc.ca.

36 Katherine Lippel, Karen Messing, Samuel Vézina, and Pascale

Prud'homme, "Conciliation travail et vie personnelle," in *Enquête québécoise sur des conditions de travail, d'emploi, de santé et de sécurité du travail(EQCOTESST)* ed. Michel Vézina, Esther Cloutier, Susan Stock, et al. (Quebec: Institut national de santé publique du Québec and Institut de la statistique du Québec—Institut de recherche Robert-Sauvé en santé et sécurité du travail, 2011), chapter 3.

37   Donna Mergler and Nicole Vézina, "Dysmenorrhea and Cold Exposure," *Journal of Reproductive Medicine* 30,2 (1985), 106–11; Karen Messing, Marie-Josèphe Saurel-Cubizolles, Madeleine Bourgine, and Monique Kaminski, "Menstrual-Cycle Characteristics and Work Conditions of Workers in Poultry Slaughterhouses and Canneries," *Scandinavian Journal of Work, Environment & Health* 18,5 (1992), 302–309; C.-C. Lin, C.-N. Huang, Y.-H. Hwang, et al., "Shortened Menstrual Cycles in LCD Manufacturing Workers," *Occupational Medicine* 63,1 (2013), 45–52; France Tissot and Karen Messing, "Perimenstrual Symptoms and Working Conditions among Hospital Workers in Quebec," *American Journal of Indistrial Medicine* 27,4 (1995), 511–22.

38   Lorraine Greaves, "We Don't Know What We Don't Know: Advocating for Women's Health Research," in *Personal & Political: Stories from the Women's Health Movement, 1960–2010,* ed. Lorraine Greaves (Toronto: Second Story Press, 2018), 347–67.

39   Stacey Ritz, David Antle, Jule Côté, et al., "First Steps for Integrating Sex and Gender Considerations into Basic Experimental Biomedical Research," *FASEB Journal* 28,1 (2014), 4–13; Robert N. Hughes, "Sex Still Matters: Has the Prevalence of Male-Only Studies of Drug Effects on Rodent Behaviour Changed during the Past Decade?," *Behavioural Pharmacology* 30,1 (2019), 95–99.

40   Yoshimitsu Inoue, Yoshiko Tanaka, Kaori Omori, et al., "Sex- and Menstrual Cycle-Related Differences in Sweating and Cutaneous Blood Flow in Response to Passive Heat Exposure," *European Journal of Applied Physiology* 94,3 (2005), 323–32.

41   Briefly reviewed in Blanca Romero-Moraleda, Juan Del Coso, Jorge Gutiérrez-Hellín, et al., "The Influence of the Menstrual Cycle on Muscle Strength and Power Performance," *Journal of Human Kinetics* 68 (2019), 123–33.

42   Robert N. Hughes, "Sex Does Matter: Comments on the Prevalence

of Male-Only Investigations of Drug Effects on Rodent Behaviour," *Behavioural Pharmacology* 18,7 (2007), 583–89.

43   Theresa M. Wizemann and Mary-Lou Pardue, eds., *Exploring the Biological Contributions to Human Health: Does Sex Matter?* (Washington, DC: National Academies Press, 2001).

44   Michael Gochfeld, "Sex Differences in Human and Animal Toxicology," *Toxicologic Pathology* 45,1 (2017), 172–89, doi: 10.1177/0192623316677327.

45   Donna Mergler, "Neurotoxic Exposures and Effects: Gender and Sex Matter! Hänninen Lecture 2011," *Neurotoxicology* 33,4 (2012), 644–51, doi: 10.1016/j.neuro.2012.05.009; Ritz, Antle, Côté, et al., "First Steps for Integrating Sex and Gender Considerations."

46   Teresa G. Valencaka, Anne Osterriederb, and Tim J. Schulz, "Sex Matters: The Effects of Biological Sex on Adipose Tissue Biology and Energy Metabolism," *Redox Biology* 12 (August 2017), 806–13.

47   Nobuko Hashiguchi, Yue Feng, and Yutaka Tochihara, "Gender Differences in Thermal Comfort and Mental Performance at Different Vertical Air Temperatures," *European Journal of Applied Physiology* 109,1 (2010), 41–48, doi: 10.1007/s00421-009-1158-7.

48   Tom Y. Chang and Agne Kajackaite, "Battle for the Thermostat: Gender and the Effect of Temperature on Cognitive Performance," *PLoS One* 15,5 (2019), e0216362, doi: 10.1371/journal.pone.0216362.

49   C. Noel Bairey Merz, Leslee J. Shaw, Steven E. Reis, et al., "Insights from the NHLBI-Sponsored Women's Ischemia Syndrome Evaluation (WISE) Study Part II: Gender Differences in Presentation, Diagnosis, and Outcome with Regard to Gender-Based Pathophysiology of Atherosclerosis and Macrovascular and Microvascular Coronary Disease," *Journal of the American College of Cardiology* 47,3 suppl. (February 2006), S21–29, doi: 10.1016/j.jacc.2004.12.

50   Rachel Cox and Karen Messing, "Legal and Biological Perspectives on Selection Tests: A Post-Meiorin Examination," *Windsor Yearbook of Access to Justice* 24 (2006), 23–53.

51   Karen Messing and Joan Stevenson, "Women in Procrustean Beds: Strength Testing and the Workplace," *Gender Work & Organization* 3,3 (1996), 156–67.

52   Julie Courville, Nicole Vézina, and Karen Messing, "Comparison of the Work Activity of Two Mechanics: A Woman and a Man," *International Journal of Industrial Ergonomics* 7,2 (1991), 163–74.

53   See also chapter 5 in my 2014 book *Pain and Prejudice.*

54   International Labour Office, "The Prohibition of Women's Night
     Work in Industry: Current Thinking and Practice," in *General Survey
     of the Reports Concerning the Night Work (Women) Convention, 1919
     (No. 4), the Night Work (Women) Convention (Revised), 1934 (No. 41),
     the Night Work (Women) convention (Revised), 1948 (No. 89), and the
     Protocol of 1990 to the Night Work (Women) Convention (Revised), 1948,*
     ed. ILO (Geneva, International Labour Office, 2009), www.ilo.org.

55   M. Sun, W. Feng, F. Wang, et al., "Meta-Analysis on Shift Work and
     Risks of Specific Obesity Types," *Obesity Reviews* 19,1 (2018), 20–48.

56   Jeanette Therming Jørgensen, Sashia Karlsen, Leslie Stayner, et al.,
     "Shift Work and Overall and Cause-Specific Mortality in the Danish
     Nurse Cohort," *Scandinavian Journal of Work, Environment & Health*
     43,2 (2017), 117–26.

57   Cox and Messing, "Legal and Biological Perspectives on Selection
     Tests."

58   Kaye N. Ballantyne, Manfred Kayser, and J. Anton Grootegoed,
     "Sex and Gender Issues in Competitive Sports: Investigation of a
     Historical Case Leads to a New Viewpoint," *British Journal of Sports
     Medicine* 46,8 (2012), 614–17.

59   Anne Fausto-Sterling, "Bare Bones of Sex: Part 1—Sex and Gender,"
     Signs 30,2 (2005), 1491–527; Hana Brzobohatá, Vaclav Krajíček,
     Zdenek Horák, and Jana Velemínská, "Sexual Dimorphism of the
     Human Tibia through Time: Insights into Shape Variation Using
     a Surface-Based Approach," *PLoS One* 11,11 (2016), e0166461, doi:
     10.1371/journal.pone.0166461.

60   Actually, speaking as a former geneticist, it is nonsense to charac-
     terize people's ethnic origins as such-and-such-a-percent European,
     Asian, etc., based on their DNA, since each continent already is
     composed of migrants from many places, and since geographical
     spaces can only be characterized by the frequencies of certain forms
     ("alleles") of genes, rather than their absolute presence or absence.
     Individuals by definition cannot have a frequency of a particular
     allele, because they only have two for each gene.

6. Re-engineering women's work

1 . Jeanne M. Stellman, *Women's Work, Women's Health* (New York: Pantheon, 1978).

2 Quebec, *S-2.1—Act Respecting Occupational Health and Safety*, Articles 40 and 46, LégisQuébec, http://legisquebec.gouv.qc.ca.

3 Agathe Croteau, Sylvie Marcoux, and Chantal Brisson, "Work Activity in Pregnancy, Preventive Measures, and the Risk of Preterm Delivery," *American Journal of Epidemiology* 166,8 (2007), 951–65; Agathe Croteau, Sylvie Marcoux, and Chantal Brisson, "Work Activity in Pregnancy, Preventive Measures, and the Risk of Delivering a Small for Gestational Age Infant," *American Journal of Public Health* 96,5 (2006), 846–55.

4 See chapter 11 of my 2014 book *Pain and Prejudice*.

5 There are other "schools" of ergonomics that put more emphasis on design of the physical elements of work situations, and less emphasis on social analysis and exchanges with workers.

6 Fabien Coutarel, Sandrine Caroly, Nicole Vézina, and François Daniellou, "Operational Leeway and Power to Act: Theoretical Issues of Ergonomics Intervention," *Le travail humain* 78,1 (2015), 9–29.

7 Marie St-Vincent, Nicole Vézina, Marie Bellemare, et al., *Ergonomic Intervention* (BookBaby, 2011).

8 Catherine Teiger, "« Les femmes aussi ont un cerveau ! » Le travail des femmes en ergonomie : réflexions sur quelques paradoxes," *Travailler* 1,15 (2006), 71–130, doi: 10.3917/trav.015.0071.

9 Christian Demers, Nicole Vézina, and Karen Messing, "Le travail en présence de rayonnements ionisants dans des laboratoires universi- taires," *Radioprotection* 26,2 (1991), 387–95.

10 Teiger, "« Les femmes aussi ont un cerveau ! »"

11 Mergler, Brabant, Vézina, and Messing, "The Weaker Sex?"; Donna Mergler and Nicole Vézina, "Dysmenorrhea and Cold Exposure," *Journal of Reproductive Medicine* 30,2 (1985), 106–11.

12 Donna Mergler, Nicole Vézina, and Annette Beauvais, "Warts among Workers in Poultry Slaughterhouses," *Scandinavian Journal of Work, Environment & Health* 8, suppl. 1 (1982), 180–84.

13 For a graphic account of the speed of an American food processing line, see: Vanesa Ribas, *On the Line: Slaughterhouse Lives and the*

Making of the New South (Oakland, CA: University of California Press, 2016).

14   Nicole Vézina, Johanne Prévost, Alain Lajoie, and Yves Beauchamp, "Élaboration d'une formation à l'affilage des couteaux : Le travail d'un collectif, travailleurs et ergonomes" [Preparation of training in knife sharpening: A collective effort by workers and ergonomists], PISTES 1,1 (1999), doi: 10.4000/pistes.3838.

15   Mergler, Brabant, Vézina, and Messing, "The Weaker Sex?"

16   Nicole Vézina, Julie Courville, and Lucie Geoffrion,"Problèmes musculo-squelettiques, caractéristiques des postes de travailleurs et des postes de travailleuses sur une chaîne de découpe de dinde," in *Invisible: Issues in Women's Occupational Health and Safety / Invisible: La santé des travailleuses,* ed. Karen Messing, Barbara Neis, and Lucie Dumais (Charlottetown, PE: Gynergy Books), 29–61.

17   Nicole Vézina and Julie Courville, "Integration of Women into Traditionally Masculine Jobs," *Women and Health* 18,3 (1992), 97–118.

18   Julie Courville, Nicole Vézina, and Karen Messing, "Analyse des facteurs ergonomiques pouvant entraîner l'exclusion des femmes du tri des colis postaux," *Le travail humain* 55 (1992), 119–34.

19   Niklas Krause, John W. Lynch, George A. Kaplan, et al., "Standing at Work and Progression of Carotid Atherosclerosis," *Scandinavian Journal of Work, Environment & Health* 26,3 (2000), 227–36, doi: 10.5271/sjweh.536; David Antle, Nicole Vézina, Karen Messing, and Julie Côté, "Development of Discomfort and Vascular and Muscular Changes during a Prolonged Standing Task," *Occupational Ergonomics* 11,1 (2013), 21–33; Karen Messing, France Tissot, and Susan Stock, "Distal Lower Extremity Pain and Working Postures in the Quebec Population," *American Journal of Public Health* 98,4 (2008), 705–13.

20   Société des Casinos du Québec, 2019 QCTAT 5726 (CanLII), www.canlii.org.

21   Thomas R. Waters and Robert B. Dick, "Evidence of Health Risks Associated with Prolonged Standing at Work and Intervention Effectiveness," *Rehabilitation Nursing* 40,3 (2015), 148–65.

7. Looking the dragon in the face

1   For example: Hélène Camirand, Issouf Traoré, and Jimmy Baulne, *L'Enquête québécoise sur la santé de la population, 2014–2015 : pour en*

savoir plus sur la santé des Québécois. Résultats de la deuxième édition (Quebec: Institut de la statistique du Québec, 2016), chapter 21.

2   France Tissot, Karen Messing, and Susan Stock, "Studying Relations between Low Back Pain and Working Postures among Those Who Stand and Those Who Sit Most of the Work Day," *Ergonomics* 52,11 (2009), 1402–18.

3   Karen Messing, Susan Stock, and France Tissot, "Work Exposures and Musculoskeletal Disorders: How the Treatment of Gender and Sex in Population-Based Surveys Can Affect Detection of Exposure-Effect Relationships," in *What a Difference Sex and Gender Make in Health Research: A CIHR Institute of Gender and Health Casebook*, ed. Institute of Gender and Health (Ottawa: Canadian Institutes of Health Research, 2012), 42–49, www.cihr-irsc.gc.ca.

4   Four cases:
Société des Casinos du Québec, 2019 QCTAT 5726 (CanLII), www.canlii.org.
Librairie Renaud-Bray inc. c. Tribunal administratif du travail, 2018 QCCS 776 (CanLII), www.canlii.org.
Emma Hinchliffe, "Walmart Set to Pay $65 Million Over Making Cashiers Stand," *Fortune,* October 14, 2018, https://fortune.com.
Kilby v. CVS Pharmacy, Inc., Supreme Court of California, 2016, https://law.justia.com.

5   Ana Maria Seifert, Karen Messing, and Lucie Dumais, "Star Wars and Strategic Defense Initiatives: Work Activity and Health Symptoms of Unionized Bank Tellers during Work Reorganization," *International Journal of Health Services* 27,3 (1997), 455–77.

6   Karen Messing, Ana Maria Seifert, and Evelin Escalona, "The 120-Second Minute: Using Analysis of Work Activity to Prevent Psychological Distress among Elementary School Teachers," *Journal of Occupational Health Psychology* 2,1 (1997), 45–62.

7   Ana Maria Seifert, Karen Messing, and Diane Elabidi, "Analyse des communications et du travail des préposées à l'accueil d'un hôpital pendant la restructuration des services," *Recherches féministes* 12,2 (1999), 85–108.

8   Katherine Lippel, "Compensation for Musculoskeletal Disorders in Quebec: Systemic Discrimination against Women Workers?," *International Journal of Health Services* 33,2 (2003), 253–81.

9   Ana Maria Seifert, Karen Messing, Céline Chatigny, and Jessica

Riel, "Precarious Employment Conditions Affect Work Content in Education and Social Work: Results of Work Analyses," *International Journal of Law and Psychiatry* 30,4–5 (2007), 299–310.

10   Johanne Prévost and Karen Messing, "Stratégies de conciliation d'un horaire de travail variable avec des responsabilités familiales," *Le travail humain* 64 (2001), 119–43. For a more detailed description of our studies of work-family articulation, see also chapter 7 of my 2014 book *Pain and Prejudice.*

11   Ana Maria Seifert and Karen Messing, "Looking and Listening in a Technical World: Effects of Discontinuity in Work Schedules on Nurses' Work Activity," *PISTES* 6,1 (2004), https://journals.openedition.org.

12   Béatrice Barthe, Karen Messing, and Lydia Abbas, "Strategies Used by Women Workers to Reconcile Family Responsibilities with Atypical Work Schedules in the Service Sector," *Work* 40 suppl. (2011), S47–58.

13   Karen Messing, Martin Chadoin, Isabelle Feillou, et al., "Soignantes ou unités interchangeables? Repenser les horaires de travail," *Le Devoir*, May 22, 2020, www.ledevoir.com.

14   Karen Messing, France Tissot, Vanessa Couture, and Stephanie Bernstein, "Strategies for Work/Life Balance of Women and Men with Variable and Unpredictable Work Hours in the Retail Sales Sector in Québec, Canada," *New Solutions: A Journal of Environmental and Occupational Health Policy* 24,2 (2014), 171–94.

15   Daycare is government-supported in Quebec, so grocery store workers would in theory have had access to it.

16   Institut de la Statistique du Québec (ISQ), "Le marché du travail et les parents" (Quebec: ISQ, 2010), table 2.1, www.stat.gouv.qc.ca.

17   Mélanie Lefrançois is now a professor at the Department of Organization and Human Resources, UQAM.

18   Mélanie Lefrançois, Johanne Saint-Charles, and Karen Messing, "Travailler la nuit comme stratégie pour augmenter sa marge de manœuvre pour concilier travail et horaires atypiques : le cas d'un service de nettoyage dans le secteur des transports," *Revue Relations Industrielles* 72,1 (2017), 99–124.

19   Mélanie Lefrançois, Karen Messing, and Johanne Saint-Charles, "Time Control, Job Execution and Information Access: Work/Family Strategies in the Context of Low-Wage Work and 24/7 Schedules," *Community, Work and Family* 20,5 (2017), 600–622.

20   Gouvernement de France, "La loi pour l'égalité réelle entre les femmes et les hommes" [Law for true equality between women and men], May 15, 2017, www.gouvernement.fr.

21   Lippel, "Compensation for Musculoskeletal Disorders in Quebec"; Katherine Lippel, "Workers' Compensation and Stress: Gender and Access to Compensation," *International Journal of Law and Psychiatry* 22,1 (1999), 79–89, doi: 10.1016/s0160-2527(98)00019-3.

22   Katherine Lippel and Karen Messing, "A Gender Perspective on Work, Regulation and Their Effects on Women's Health, Safety and Well-Being" in *Safety or Profit?: International Studies in Governance, Change and the Work Environment,* ed. Theo Nichols and David Walters (New York: Baywood, 2014), 33–48.

23   Pamela Astudillo, Carlos Ibarra, and Julia Medel, *Guía de Formación en Ergonomía y Género para dirigentes sindicales* (Santiago, Chile: Instituto de Salud Pública de Chile, 2015), www.researchgate.net.

24   Cox and Messing, "Legal and Biological Perspectives on Selection Tests."

25   Lefrançois, Messing, and Saint-Charles, "Time Control, Job Execution and Information Access."

26   A reference to Simone de Beauvoir, *The Second Sex,* trans. Constance Borde and Sheila Malovany-Chevallier (New York: Alfred A. Knopf, 2009).

27   Stephanie Bernstein and Mathilde Valentini, "Working Time and Family Life: Looking at the Intersection of Labour and Family Law in Québec," *Journal of Law and Equality* 14,1 (2018).

28   Agence nationale pour l'amélioration des conditions de travail (ANACT), *Un kit pour prévenir le sexisme* (Lyon, France, 2016), www.egalite-femmes-hommes.gouv.fr.

8. Feminist ergonomic intervention with a feminist employer

1   Ana Maria Seifert and Karen Messing, "Cleaning Up after Globalization: An Ergonomic Analysis of Work Activity of Hotel Cleaners," *Antipode* 38,3 (2006), 557–77.

2   Céline Chatigny, Karen Messing, Eve Laperrière, and Marie-Christine Thibault, "Battle Fatigue: Identifying Stressors That Affect Counsellors in Women's Shelters," *Canadian Woman Studies* 24,1

(2005), 139–44; Marie-Christine Thibault, Eve Laperrière, Céline Chatigny, and Karen Messing, *Des intervenantes* à *tout faire : analyse du travail en maison d'hébergement* (Montreal: Service aux collectivités, Université du Québec à Montréal, 2003).

3   Catherine Teiger and Colette Bernier, "Ergonomic Analysis of Work Activity of Data Entry Clerks in the Computerized Service Sector Can Reveal Unrecognized Skills," *Women and Health* 18,3 (1992), 67–77.

4   This is why ergonomists generally portray ourselves as positivist scientists, like chemists or physicists, who formulate hypotheses and produce evidence that supports or invalidates them. The founders of the type of ergonomics taught at Conservatoire national des arts et métiers (CNAM) were two physicians, an engineer and a psychologist, and they thought of their ergonomics as a biomedical and not a social science. But this view was later questioned by a founder, Dr. Alain Wisner, who described it as closer to anthropology or ethnography. Both positivist and constructivist traditions still co-exist in ergonomics, but I have to admit that, trained in biology, I am more of a positivist.

5   Karen Messing, Nancy Guberman, Céline Chatigny, et al., *Analyse du travail dans les maisons d'hébergement pour femmes victimes de violence conjugale : approche en ergonomie et en travail social* (Montreal: Université du Québec à Montréal, 2005).

6   The difference between average time and median time can occur when one or two events in an average take an exceptionally long (or short) time. For example, some one-on-one interviews could last a half-hour before being interrupted, so the average time is longer than the median time.

7   This reminded me of my observations in a retail store where smokers were the only workers allowed to take sitting breaks, because their manager, a smoker himself, understood that smoking was a physiological necessity. (He didn't have the same empathetic understanding of working postures, so the non-smoking workers had no breaks to sit down.) I wondered whether smoking could sometimes be a positive occupational health determinant!

8   Céline Chatigny, "Devising Work Schedules for a Collective: Favouring Intergenerational Collaboration among Counsellors in a Shelter for Female Victims of Conjugal Violence," *Work* 40 suppl. (2011), S101–110.

9   Susan J. Lambert, Julia R. Henly, Michael Schoeny, and Meghan Jarpe, "Increasing Schedule Predictability in Hourly Jobs: Results from a Randomized Experiment in a U.S. Retail Firm," *Work and Occupations* 46,2 (2019), 176–226, doi: 10.1177/0730888418823241.

10   Vérificateur général du Québec, *Rapport du Vérificateur général du Québec à l'Assemblée nationale pour l'année 2019–2020 : Commission des normes, de l'équité, de la santé et de la sécurité du travail. Audit de performance prévention en santé et en sécurité du travail* (Québec: Vérificateur général du Québec, 2019), www.vgq.qc.ca.

9. Solidarity

1   Before I was hired as a professor, I had lectured on biology in the course.

2   « Je suis blessée dans mon orgueil de femme! »

3   See chapter 8 of my 2014 book *Pain and Prejudice* for the story of how Donna and I realized we could head a team without necessarily including a man in the leadership, and how our funding agency reacted.

4   Karen Messing, "La place des femmes dans les priorités de recherche en santé au travail au Québec," *Relations Industrielles / Industrial Relations* 57,4 (2002), 660–86.

5   www.relais-femmes.qc.ca

6   www.iref.uqam.ca

7   Syndicat des professeurs et professeures de l'Université du Québec à Montréal (SPUQ), "Conventions collectives : Convention des professeures et des professeurs signée le 20 décembre 2018, en vigueur jusqu'au 31 mai 2022," Article 29 : Accès à l'égalité pour les femmes, https://spuq.uqam.ca.

8   Shelia H. Zahm and Aaron Blair, "Occupational Cancer among Women: Where Have We Been and Where Are We Going?," *American Journal of Industrial Medicine* 44,6 (2003), 565–75; Isabelle Niedhammer, Marie-Josèphe Saurel-Cubizolles, Michèle Piciotti, and Sébastien Bonenfant, "How Is Sex Considered in Recent Epidemiological Publications on Occupational Risks?," *Occupational and Environmental Medicine* 57,8 (2000), 521–27.

9   Messing, "La place des femmes dans les priorités de recherche."

10   Karen Messing and Sophie Boutin, "La reconnaissance des conditions

difficiles dans les emplois des femmes et les instances gouverne-
mentales en santé et en sécurité du travail," *Relations Industrielles /
Industrial Relations* 52,2 (1997), 333–62.

11 Katherine Lippel, "Workers' Compensation and Psychological Stress
Claims in North American Law: A Microcosmic Model of Systemic
Discrimination," *International Journal of Law and Psychiatry* 12,1
(1989), 41–70.

12 Aaron Derfel, "Job-Safety Rules Are Failing Women, UQAM Study
Says," *Montreal Gazette*, March 18, 1996, 1.

13 Patrice Duguay, François Hébert, and Paul Massicotte, "Les indicateurs de lésions indemnisées en santé et en sécurité du travail au
Québec : des différences selon le sexe," in *Comptes rendus du congrès
de la Société d'ergonomie de langue française(SELF)*, vol. 6 (Montreal:
SELF, 2001), 65–69.

14 Canadian Institutes of Health Research (CIHR), "CIHR Research
Chairs in Gender, Work and Health," www.cihr-irsc.gc.ca.

15 Pascale Prud'homme, Marc-Antoine Busque, Patrice Duguay, and
Daniel Côté, *Immigrant Workers and OHS in Québec State of Knowledge
from Published Statistical Surveys and Available Data Sources* (Montreal:
Institut de Recherche Robert-Sauvé en Santé et en Sécurité du
Travail, 2017), www.irsst.qc.ca.

16 Unfortunately a casualty of the Conservative Harper government not
restored by the succeeding Liberals.

17 Karen Messing, *Occupational Health and Safety Concerns of Canadian
Women: A Background Paper* (Ottawa: Labour Canada, 1991).

18 Karen Messing, Barbara Neis, and Lucie Dumais, eds., *Invisible: Issues
in Women's Occupational Health and Safety / Invisible : La santé des
travailleuses* (Charlottetown, PE: Gynergy Books, 1995).

19 Karen Messing and Donna Mergler, eds., *Women's Occupational and
Environmental Health* (special issue), *Environmental Research* 101,2
(2006), 147–286.

20 Greaves, "We Don't Know What We Don't Know."

21 Joy Johnson, Zena Sharman, Bilkis Vissandjée, and Donna E. Stewart,
"Does a Change in Health Research Funding Policy Related to the
Integration of Sex and Gender Have an Impact?," *PLoS One* 9,6
(2014), e99900, doi: 10.1371/journal.pone.0099900; Zena Sharman
and Joy Johnson, "Towards the Inclusion of Gender and Sex in Health
Research and Funding: An Institutional Perspective," *Social Science*

& *Medicine* 74,11 (2012), 1812–6, doi: 10.1016/j.socscimed.2011.08.039; Cara Tannenbaum, Lorraine Greaves, and Ian D. Graham, "Why Sex and Gender Matter in Implementation Research," *BMC Medical Research Methodology* 16,1 (2016), 145, doi: 10.1186/s12874-016-0247-7; Annie Duchesne, Cara Tannenbaum, and Gillian Einstein, "Funding Agency Mechanisms to Increase Sex and Gender Analysis," *Lancet* 389,10070 (2017), 699, doi: 10.1016/s0140-6736(17)0343-4.

22 Despite the name, the book included analyses from both law and ergonomics, covering such subjects as inadequate rehabilitation practices and unfairness in compensation for injured women workers.

23 Karen Messing and Piroska Östlin, *Gender Equality, Work and Health: A Review of the Evidence* (Geneva: World Health Organization, 2006), www.who.int.

24 Linda M. Pottern, Shelia Hoar Zahm, and Susan S. Sieber, "Occupational Cancer among Women: A Conference Overview," *Journal of Occupational Medicine* 36,8 (1994), 809–813.

25 Even in our current very conservative Quebec government, the governing party was forced to include 40% female candidates (as were the other three major parties) and eventually 50% women ministers.

10. Science and the second body

1 Vilma Hunt, *Work and the Health of Women* (Boca Raton, FL: CRC Press, 1979); Jeanne M. Stellman, *Women's Work, Women's Health: Myths and Realities* (New York: Pantheon, 1978); Pottern, Zahm, and Sieber, "Occupational Cancer among Women."

2 Messing, *One-Eyed Science.*

3 Isabelle Niedhammer, Marie-Josèphe Saurel-Cubizolles, Michèle Piciotti, and Sébastien Bonenfant, "How Is Sex Considered in Recent Epidemiological Publications on Occupational Risks?," *Occupational and Environmental Medicine* 57,8 (2000), 521–27.

4 Karin Hohenadel, Priyanka Raj, Paul A. Demers, et al., "The Inclusion of Women in Studies of Occupational Cancer: A Review of the Epidemiologic Literature from 1991–2009," *American Journal of Industrial Medicine* 58,3 (2015), 276–81; Olivier Betansedi, Patricia Vaca Vasquez, and Émilie Counil, "A Comprehensive Approach of the Gender Bias in Occupational Cancer Epidemiology: A Systematic

Review of Lung Cancer Studies (2003–2014)," *American Journal of Industrial Medicine* 61,5 (2018), 372–82, doi: 10.1002/ajim.22823.

5   Annaliese K. Beery and Irving Zucker, "Sex Bias in Neuroscience and Biomedical Research," *Neuroscience & Biobehavioral Reviews* 35,3 (2011), 565–72; Gochfeld, "Sex Differences in Human and Animal Toxicology."

6   Rosemary M. Bowler, Donna Mergler, Stephen S. Rauch, and Russell P. Bowler, "Stability of Psychological Impairment: Two Year Follow-Up of Former Microelectronics Workers' Affective and Personality Disturbance," *Women and Health* 18,1 (1992), 27–48. According to Donna Mergler, women are 15%–20% of those exposed to solvents at work.

7   Donna Mergler, "Les défis de transfert de connaissances et de l'intégration du sexe et du genre," invited lecture, CINBIOSE team on integrated knowledge transfer, April 16, 2019.

8   Sabrina Llopa, Maria-Jose Lopez-Espinosa, Marisa Rebagliatob, and Ferran Ballester, "Gender Differences in the Neurotoxicity of Metals in Children," *Toxicology* 311,1–2 (2013), 3–12.

9   Holly O. Witteman, Michael Hendricks, Sharon Straus, and Cara Tannenbaum, "Are Gender Gaps Due to Evaluations of the Applicant or the Science?: A Natural Experiment at a National Funding Agency," *Lancet* 393,7439 (2019), 531–40.

10   Markus Helmer, Manuel Schottdorf, Andreas Neef, and Demian Battaglia, "Gender Bias in Scholarly Peer Review," *eLife* 6 (2017), e21718, doi: 10.7554/eLife.21718; Charles W. Fox and C.E. Timothy Paine, "Gender Differences in Peer Review Outcomes and Manuscript Impact at Six Journals of Ecology and Evolution," *Ecology and Evolution* 9,6 (2019), 3599–619.

11   Helen Shen, "Inequality Quantified: Mind the Gender Gap," *Nature* 495 (March 7, 2013), 22–24.

12   Lippel, "Compensation for Musculoskeletal Disorders in Quebec." The appeal level is the only level where the success rate can be measured, since data on claims heard at lower levels are not available.

13   Ola Leijon, Emil Lindahl, Kjell Torén, et al., "First-Time Decisions Regarding Work Injury Annuity Due to Occupational Disease: A Gender Perspective," *Occupational and Environmental Medicine* 71,2 (2014), 147–53.

14   Lippel, "Compensation for Musculoskeletal Disorders in Quebec."

15 Katherine Lippel, Marie-Claire Lefebvre, Chantal Schmidt, and Joseph Caron, *Managing Claims or Caring for Claimants: Effects of the Compensation Proces on the Health of Injured Workers* (Montreal: Université du Québec à Montréal, Service aux collectivités, 2007), 45.

16 Lippel, Lefebvre, Schmidt, and Caron, *Managing Claims or Caring for Claimants*, 30.

17 Karina Lauenborg Møller, Charlotte Brauer, Sigurd Mikkelsen, et al., "Copenhagen Airport Cohort: Air Pollution, Manual Baggage Handling and Health," *BMJ Open* 7,5 (2017), e012651, doi: 10.1136/bmjopen-2016- 012651; Henrik Koblauch, "Low Back Load in Airport Baggage Handlers," *Danish Medical Journal* 63,4 (2016), 1–35, https://ugeskriftet.dk; Alireza Tafazzol, Samin Aref, Majid Mardani, et al., "Epidemiological and Biomechanical Evaluation of Airline Baggage Handling," *International Journal of Occupational Safety and Ergonomics* 22,2 (2016), 218–27, doi: 10.1080/10803548.2015.1126457; Sane Pagh Møller, Charlotte Brauer, Sigurd Mikkelsen, et al., "Risk of Subacromial Shoulder Disorder in Airport Baggage Handlers: Combining Duration and Intensity of Musculoskeletal Shoulder Loads," *Ergonomics* 61,4 (2018), 576–87.

18 Valérie Simonneaux and Thibault Bahougne, "A Multi-Oscillatory Circadian System Times Female Reproduction," *Frontiers in Endocrinology* 6 (2015), 157, doi: 10.3389/fendo.2015.00157.

19 Donna Mergler and Nicole Vézina, "Dysmenorrhea and Cold Exposure," *Journal of Reproductive Medicine* 30,2 (1985), 106–11; Karen Messing, Marie-Josèphe Saurel-Cubizolles, Madeleine Bourgine, and Monique Kaminski, "Factors Associated with Dysmenorrhea among Workers in French Poultry Slaughterhouses and Canneries," *Journal of Occupational Medicine* 35,5 (1993), 493–500; Tze Pin Ng, Swee Cheng Foo, and Theresa Yoong, "Menstrual Function in Workers Exposed to Toluene," *British Journal of Industrial Medicine* 49,11 (1992), 799–803.

20 Kuntala Lahiri-Dutt and Kathryn Robinson, "'Period Problems' at the Coalface," *Feminist Review* 89 (2008), 102–121.

21 Priya Kannan, Stanley Winser, Ravindra Goonetilleke, and Gladys Cheing, "Ankle Positions Potentially Facilitating Greater Maximal Contraction of Pelvic Floor Muscles: A Systematic Review and Meta-Analysis," *Disability and Rehabilitation* 41,21 (2019), 2483–91.

22 Cara Kelly, "NASA's Spacesuit Issue Is All Too Familiar for Working Women," *USA Today*, March 28, 2019, www.usatoday.com.

23 For a well-documented, fascinating account of sexism in design, I recommend: Caroline Criado Perez, *Invisible Women: Exposing Data Bias in a World Designed for Men* (London: Chatto & Windus, 2019).

24 Ana Maria Seifert and Karen Messing, "Looking and Listening in a Technical World: Effects of Discontinuity in Work Schedules on Nurses' Work Activity," PISTES 6,1 (2004), doi: 10.4000/pistes.3285.

25 Cassidy R. Sugimoto, Yong-Yeol Ahn, Elise Smith, et al., "Factors Affecting Sex-Related Reporting in Medical Research: A Cross-Disciplinary Bibliometric Analysis," *Lancet* 393,10171 (2019), 550–59; Sarah Hawkes, Fariha Haseen, and Hajer Aounallah Skhiri, "Measurement and Meaning: Reporting Sex in Health Research," *Lancet* 393,10171 (2019), 497–99, doi: 10.1016/S0140-6736(19)30283-1.

11. Understanding women's pain

1   Stephanie Premji, Karen Messing, and Katherine Lippel, "Broken English, Broken Bones?: Mechanisms Linking Language Proficiency and Occupational Health in a Montreal Garment Factory," *International Journal of Health Services* 38,1 (2008), 1–19.

2   Stephanie Premji, Katherine Lippel, and Karen Messing, "« On travaille à la seconde! » Rémunération à la pièce et santé et sécurité du travail dans une perspective qui tient compte de l'ethnicité et du genre," *PISTES* 10,1 (2008), doi: 10.4000/pistes.2181.

3   Stephanie Premji, Patrick Duguay, Karen Messing, and Katherine Lippel, "Are Immigrants, Ethnic and Linguistic Minorities Over-represented in Jobs with a High Level of Compensated Risk?: Results from a Montréal, Canada Study Using Census and Workers' Compensation Data," *American Journal of Industrial Medicine* 53,9 (2010), 875–85.

4   France Tissot, Susan Stock, and Nektaria Nicolakakis, *Portrait des troubles musculo-squelettiques d'origine non traumatique liés au travail : résultats de L'enquête québécoise sur la santé de la population, 2014–2015* (Québec, Institut national de santé publique, 2020), www.inspq.qc.ca.

5   Marie-Eve Major and Nicole Vézina, "The Organization of Working Time: Developing an Understanding and Action Plan to Promote Workers' Health in a Seasonal Work Context," *New Solutions: A Journal of Occupational and Environmental Health Policy* 27,3 (2017), 403–423, doi: 10.1177/1048291117725712.

6   Nicole Vézina, Daniel Tierney, and Karen Messing, "When Is Light Work Heavy?: Components of the Physical Workload of Sewing Machine Operators Which May Lead to Health Problems," *Applied Ergonomics* 23,4 (1992), 268–76.

7   Courville, Vézina, and Messing, "Analyse des facteurs ergonomiques"; Katherine Lippel, Karen Messing, Susan Stock, and Nicole Vézina, "La preuve de la causalité et l'indemnisation des lésions attribuables au travail répétitif : rencontre des sciences de la santé et du droit," *Windsor Yearbook of Access to Justice* XVII (1999), 35–86.

8   France Tissot, Karen Messing, and Susan Stock, "Standing, Sitting and Associated Working Conditions in the Quebec Population in 1998," *Ergonomics* 48,3 (2005), 249–69; Karen Messing, Sylvie Fortin, Geneviève Rail, and Maude Randoin, "Standing Still: Why North American Workers Are Not Insisting on Seats, Despite Known Health Benefits," *International Journal of Health Services* 35,4 (2005), 745–63.

9   Jun Deokhoon, Zoe Michaleff, Venerina Johnston, and Shaun O'Leary, "Physical Risk Factors for Developing Non-specific Neck Pain in Office Workers: A Systematic Review and Meta-analysis," *International Archives of Occupational and Environmental Health* 90,5 (2017), 373–410, doi: 10.1007/s00420-017-1205-3.

10   Tim Morse, Renee Fekieta, Harriet Rubenstein, et al., "Doing the Heavy Lifting: Health Care Workers Take Back Their Backs," *New Solutions: A Journal of Occupational and Environmental Health Policy* 18,2 (2008), 207–19, doi: 10.2190/NS.18.2.j.

11   Karen Messing and Åsa Kilbom, "Standing and Very Slow Walking: Foot Pain-Pressure Threshold, Subjective Pain Experience and Work Activity," *Applied Ergonomics* 32 (2001), 81–90.

12   Yolande Lucire, "Social Iatrogenesis of the Australian Disease 'RSI,'" *Community Health Studies* 12,2 (1988), 146–50; J.L. Quintner, "The Australian RSI Debate: Stereotyping and Medicine," *Disability and Rehabilitation* 17,5 (1995), 256–62.

13   Charles V. Ford, "Somatization and Fashionable Diagnoses: Illness as a Way of Life," *Scandinavian Journal of Work, Environment & Health* 23, suppl. 3 (1997), 7–16.

14   Theo Vos, Abraham D. Flaxman, Mohsen Naghavi, et al., "Years Lived with Disability (YLDS) for 1160 Sequelae of 289 Diseases and Injuries, 1990–2010: A Systematic Analysis for the Global Burden of Disease Study, 2010," *Lancet* 380,9859 (2012), 2163–96.

15   Alessio D'Addona, Nicola Maffulli, Silvestro Formisano, and Donato
      Rosa, "Inflammation in Tendinopathy," *Surgeon* 15,5 (2017), 297–302.

16   Lars Arendt-Nielsen, Søren T. Skou, Thomas A. Nielsen, and Kristian
      K. Petersen, "Altered Central Sensitization and Pain Modulation
      in the CNS in Chronic Joint Pain," *Current Osteoporosis Reports* 13
      (2015), 225–34.

17   Kayleigh De Meulemeester, Patrick Calders, Robby De Pauw, et al.,
      "Morphological and Physiological Differences in the Upper Trapezius
      Muscle in Patients with Work-Related Trapezius Myalgia Compared
      to Healthy Controls: A Systematic Review," *Musculoskeletal Science and
      Practice* 29 (2017), 43–51.

18   Arendt-Nielsen, Skou, Nielsen, and Petersen, "Altered Central
      Sensitization and Pain Modulation."

19   Roxanne Pelletier, Karin H. Humphries, Avi Shimony, et al., "Sex-
      Related Differences in Access to Care among Patients with Premature
      Acute Coronary Syndrome," *Canadian Medical Association Journal*
      186,7 (2014), 497–504, doi: 10.1503/cmaj.131450.

20   Valérie Lederer and Michèle Rivard, "Compensation Benefits in
      a Population-Based Cohort of Men and Women on Long-Term
      Disability after Musculoskeletal Injuries: Costs, Course, Predictors,"
      Occupational and Environmental Medicine 71,11 (2014), 772–79.

21   O.A. Alabas, O.A. Tashani, G. Tabasam, and M.I. Johnson, "Gender
      Role Affects Experimental Pain Responses: A Systematic Review with
      Meta-Analysis," *European Journal of Pain* 16,9 (2012), 1211–23.

22   E.J. Bartley and R.B. Fillingim, "Sex Differences in Pain: A Brief
      Review of Clinical and Experimental Findings," *British Journal of
      Anaesthesia* 111,1 (2013), 52–58.

23   Robert E. Sorge, Josiane Mapplebeck, and Sarah Rosen, "Different
      Immune Cells Mediate Mechanical Pain Hypersensitivity in Male and
      Female Mice," *Nature Neuroscience* 18,8 (2015), 1081–83.

24   A CBC interview with Institute of Gender and Health director Cara
      Tannenbaum and researcher Jeffrey Mogil recently described this
      problem: "Sexism in Mouse Research Can Lead to Medical Harm to
      Women, Scientists Warn," CBC News, April 20, 2016, www.cbc.ca.
      See also "Of Mice and Women: Scientists Push to Fix Gender Gap
      in Lab Rats For Research," *The Current*, CBC Radio, April 20, 2016,
      www.cbc.ca.

25 Cordelia Fine, *Delusions of Gender: How Our Minds, Society, and Neurosexism Create Difference* (New York: WW Norton, 2010).

26 Camirand, Traoré, and Baulne, *L'Enquête québécoise sur la santé de la population, 2014–2015*, 185.

27 Susan Stock, Amélie Funes, Alain Delisle, et al., "Troubles Musculo-squelettiques" in *EQCOTESST*, ed. Vézina, Cloutier, Stock, et al., chapter 7.

28 Camirand, Traoré, and Baulne, *L'Enquête québécoise sur la santé de la population, 2014–2015*.

29 Susan R. Stock and France Tissot, "Are There Health Effects of Harassment in the Workplace?: A Gender-Sensitive Study of the Relationships between Work and Neck Pain," *Ergonomics* 55,2 (2012), 147–59.

30 Karen Messing, France Tissot, Susan Stock, "Distal Lower Extremity Pain and Working Postures in the Quebec Population," *American Journal of Public Health* 98,4 (2008), 705–13.

31 Karen Messing, Susan Stock, Julie Côté, and France Tissot, "Is Sitting Worse Than Static Standing?: How a Gender Analysis Can Move Us toward Understanding Determinants and Effects of Occupational Standing and Walking," *Journal of Occupational and Environmental Hygiene* 12,3 (2015), D11–17.

32 Esther Cloutier, Patrice Duguay, Samuel Vézina, and Pascale Prud'homme, "Accidents de travail," in *EQCOTESST*, ed. Vézina, Cloutier, Stock, et al., chapter 8.

33 I should note that the growth of the service sector is changing the portrait of occupational hazards, as we saw during the COVID pandemic. Now female school teachers, hospital workers, and convenience store cashiers are increasingly attacked by customers, making women much more likely than men to be physically attacked at work. And women can be subject to slips and falls in cleaning, food service, and other occupations, while men can be exposed to chronic musculoskeletal problems from prolonged standing.

34 Susan Stock, Nektaria Nicolakakis, France Tissot, et al., *Inégalités de santé au travail entre les salariés visés et ceux non visés par les mesures préventives prévues par la loi sur la santé et la sécurité du travail* (Quebec: Institut national de santé publique, 2020).

12. The technical is political

1   Mergler, Brabant, Vézina, and Messing, "The Weaker Sex?"

2   Note (for any statisticians or epidemiologists who may be reading this) that the usual tests for interactions with gender had nevertheless showed no significant multiplicative interactions, possibly because there were too many empty or near-empty cells due to the fact that men's and women's working conditions were very different from each other.

3   Karen Messing, Laura Punnett, Meg Bond, et al., "Be The Fairest of Them All: Challenges and Recommendations for the Treatment of Gender in Occupational Health Research," *American Journal of Industrial Medicine* 43,6 (2003), 618–29.

4   Michael B. Lax, "The Fetish of the Objective Finding," *New Solutions: A Journal of Occupational and Environmental Health Policy* 10,3 (2000), 237–56.

5   Pat Armstrong and Karen Messing, "Taking Gender into Account in Occupational Health Research: Continuing Tensions," *Policy and Practice in Health and Safety* 12,1 (2014), 3–16; Nancy Krieger, "Women and Social Class: A Methodological Study Comparing Individual, Household, and Census Measures as Predictors of Black/White Differences in Reproductive History," *Journal of Epidemiology and Community Health* 45,1 (1991), 35–42.

6   Stephen S. Bao, Jay M. Kapellusch, Arun Garg, et al., "Developing a Pooled Job Physical Exposure Data Set from Multiple Independent Studies: An Example of a Consortium Study of Carpal Tunnel Syndrome," *Occupational and Environmental Medicine* 72,2 (2015), 130–37.

7   Joan Eakin, "Towards a 'Standpoint' Perspective: Health and Safety in Small Workplaces from the Perspective of the Workers," *Policy and Practice in Health and Safety* 8,2 (2010), 113–27.

8   Karen Messing, "Pain and Prejudice: Does Collecting Information from the Standpoint of Exposed Workers Improve Scientific Examination of Work-Related Musculoskeletal Disorders?," *International Journal of Health Services* 46,3 (2016), 465–82.

9   Karen Messing and Jeanne M. Stellman, "Sex, Gender and Health: The Importance of Considering Mechanism," *Environmental Research* 101,2 (2006), 149–62, doi: 10.1016/j.envres.2005.03.015.

10   Stephanie Premji, "'It's Totally Destroyed Our Life': Exploring the Pathways and Mechanisms between Precarious Employment and Health and Well-Being among Immigrant Men and Women in Toronto," *International Journal of Health Services* 48,1 (2018), 106–127, doi: 10.1177/0020731417730011.

11   Martha Stanbury and Kenneth D. Rosenman, "Occupational Health Disparities: A State Public Health-Based Approach," *American Journal of Industrial Medicine* 57,5 (2014), 596–604, doi: 10.1002/ajim.22292.

12   Anu Polvinen, Mikko Laaksonen, Raija Gould, et al., "The Contribution of Major Diagnostic Causes to Socioeconomic Differences in Disability Retirement," *Scandinavian Journal of Work, Environment & Health* 40,4 (2014), 353–60, doi: 10.5271/sjweh.3411.

13   Premji, Duguay, Messing, and Lippel, "Are Immigrants, Ethnic and Linguistic Minorities Over-represented in Jobs with a High Level of Compensated Risk?"

14   Annika Härenstam, "Exploring Gender, Work and Living Conditions, and Health—Suggestions for Contextual and Comprehensive Approaches," *Scandinavian Journal of Work, Environment & Health* 35,2 (2009), 127–33.

15   Ola Leijon, Annika Härenstam, Kerstin Waldenströma, et al., "Target Groups for Prevention of Neck/Shoulder and Low Back Disorders: An Exploratory Cluster Analysis of Working and Living Conditions," *Work* 27,2 (2006), 189–204.

16   Karen Messing, Mélanie Lefrançois, and France Tissot, "Genre et statistiques : est-ce que « l'analyse de grappes » peut nous aider à comprendre la place du genre dans la recherche de solutions pour l'articulation travail-famille?," *PISTES* 18,2 (2016), doi: 10.4000/pistes.4854.

17   See their website for an overview of their actions: www.cihr-irsc.gc.ca/e/51310.html.

18   The Institute of Gender and Health is collaborating with the epidemiologist Mahée Gilbert-Ouimet on this project.

19   Hohenadel, Raj, Demers, et al., "The Inclusion of Women in Studies of Occupational Cancer."

20   Lani R. Wegrzyn, Rulla M. Tamimi, Bernard A. Rosner, et al., "Rotating Night-Shift Work and the Risk of Breast Cancer in the Nurses' Health Studies," *American Journal of Epidemiology* 186,5 (2017), 532–40, doi: 10.1093/aje/kwx140.

21   E. Garcia, P.T. Bradshaw, and E.A. Eisen, "Breast Cancer Incidence and Exposure to Metalworking Fluid in a Cohort of Female Autoworkers," *American Journal of Epidemiology* 187,3 (2018), 539–47, doi: 10.1093/aje/kwx264; James T. Brophy, Margaret M. Keith, Andrew Watterson, et al., "Breast Cancer Risk in Relation to Occupations with Exposure to Carcinogens and Endocrine Disruptors: A Canadian Case-Control Study," *Environmental Health* 11,87 (2012), doi: 10.1186/1476-069X-11-87; Per Gustavsson, Tomas Andersson, Annika Gustavsson, and Christina Reuterwall, "Cancer Incidence in Female Laboratory Employees: Extended Follow-Up of a Swedish Cohort Study," *Occupational and Environmental Medicine* 74,11 (2017), 823–26, doi: 10.1136/oemed-2016-104184.

22   P. Cocco, L. Figgs, Mustafa Dosemeci, et al., "Case-Control Study of Occupational Exposures and Male Breast Cancer," *Occupational and Environmental Medicine* 55,9 (1998), 599–604; Anne Grundy, Shelley A. Harris, Paul A. Demers, et al., "Occupational Exposure to Magnetic Fields and Breast Cancer among Canadian Men," *Cancer Medicine* 5,3 (2016), 586–96.

23   Susan Phillips, "Measuring the Health Effects of Gender," *Journal of Epidemiology and Community Health* 62,4 (2008), 368–71.

24   Peter Smith and Mieke Koehoorn, "Measuring Gender When You Don't Have a Gender Measure: Constructing a Gender Index Using Survey Data," *International Journal for Equity in Health* 15,1 (2016), 82.

25   Haining Yang, Zeyana Rivera, Sandro Jube, et al., "Programmed Necrosis Induced by Asbestos in Human Mesothelial Cells Causes High-Mobility Group Box 1 Protein Release and Resultant Inflammation," *Proceedings of the National Academy of Sciences* 107,28 (2010), 12611–16, doi: 10.1073/pnas.1006542107.

26   Greta R. Bauer, Jessica Braimoh, Ayden I. Scheim, Christoffer Dharma, "Transgender-Inclusive Measures of Sex/Gender for Population Surveys: Mixed-Methods Evaluation and Recommendations," *PLoS One* 12,5 (2017), e0178043, doi: 10.1371/journal.pone.0178043.

27   Greta R. Bauer and Ayden I. Scheim, "Methods for Analytic Intercategorical Intersectionality in Quantitative Research: Discrimination as a Mediator of Health Inequalities," *Social Science and Medicine* 226 (2019), 236–45.

28 Conference Board of Canada, *The Business Case for Women on Boards* (Ottawa: Conference Board of Canada, 2012), www.conferenceboard.ca.

29 Jessica Riel, Céline Chatigny, and Karen Messing, "On veut travailler ensemble, mais c'est difficile. Obstacles organisationnels et sociaux au travail collectif en enseignement d'un métier à prédominance masculine en formation professionnelle au secondaire au Québec," *Revue des sciences de l'éducation* 42,3 (2016), 36–68; Mélanie Lefrançois, Johanne Saint-Charles, and Jessica Riel, "Work/Family Balancing and 24/7 Work Schedules: Network Analysis of Strategies in a Transport Company Cleaning Service," *New Solutions: A Journal of Occupational and Environmental Health Policy* 27,3 (2017), 319–41, doi: 10.1177/1048291117725718.

30 Sandrine Caroly, "How Police Officers and Nurses Regulate Combined Domestic and Paid Workloads to Manage Schedules: A Gender Analysis," *Work* 40, suppl. 1 (2011), S71–82, doi: 10.3233/WOR-2011-1269.

31 Meng-Jung Chung and Mao-Jiun Wang, "Gender and Walking Speed Effects on Plantar Pressure Distribution for Adults Aged 20–60 Years," *Ergonomics* 55,2 (2012), 194–200.

32 Donna Mergler and Nicole Vézina, "Dysmenorrhea and Cold Exposure," *Journal of Reproductive Medicine* 30,2 (1985), 106–11.

33 Yoonjung Kim and Yeunhee Kwak, "Urinary Incontinence in Women in Relation to Occupational Status," *Women & Health* 57,1 (2017), 1–18, doi: 10.1080/03630242.2016.1150387.

34 Joan M. Stevenson, D.R. Greenhorn, John Timothy Bryant, et al., "Gender Differences in Performance of a Selection Test Using the Incremental Lifting Machine," *Applied Ergonomics* 27,1 (1996), 45–52.

35 Allard Dembe and Xiaoxi Yao, "Chronic Disease Risks from Exposure to Long-Hour Work Schedules over a 32-Year Period," *Journal of Occupational and Environmental Medicine* 58,9 (2016), 861–67; Jørgensen, Karlsen, Stayner, et al., "Shift Work and Overall and Cause-Specific Mortality."

36 Mergler, "Neurotoxic Exposures and Effects: Gender and Sex Matter!"

13. Going forward together

1   ". . . the redefinition of the 'normal worker' as including women—and men—with a broad range of family obligations that necessarily may interfere with work is a sine qua non for achieving work-family balance." Quoted from Stephanie Bernstein, "Addressing Work-Family Conflict in Quebec: The Gap between Policy Discourse and Legal Response," *Canadian Labour & Employment Law Journal* 20,2 (2017), 273–306. See also Bernstein and Valentini, "Working Time and Family Life."

2   Agence nationale pour l'amélioration des conditions de travail (ANACT), *Un kit pour prévenir le sexisme* (Lyon, France, 2016), www.egalite-femmes-hommes.gouv.fr.

3   Messing, "A Feminist Intervention That Hurt Women."

4   Marie Laberge, Vanessa Luong-Blanchette, Arnaud Blanchard, et al., "Impacts of Considering Sex and Gender during Intervention Studies in Occupational Health: Researchers' Perspectives," *Applied Ergonomics* 82,1 (2020), doi: 10.1016/j.apergo.2019.102960.

INDEX